VEGGIE BINGO

WINNING THE BATTLE OF INFLAMMATION IN A FUN, NATURAL, NUTRITIOUS WAY!

DR. CHRISTINE E. MAYO POWERS

PHARMD BCPS

ISBN: 978-1-54394-074-9 (print)

ISBN: 978-1-54394-075-6 (ebook)

For Bruce,
you are an amazing husband,
partner and friend.

TABLE OF CONTENTS

Have you ever needed pain relief?

Have you ever wondered if there was a way to take charge of your health? Have you wondered about inflammation and what it is doing to your body?

Then Veggie Bingo is for YOU!

Let's start a health revolution right in our kitchens!

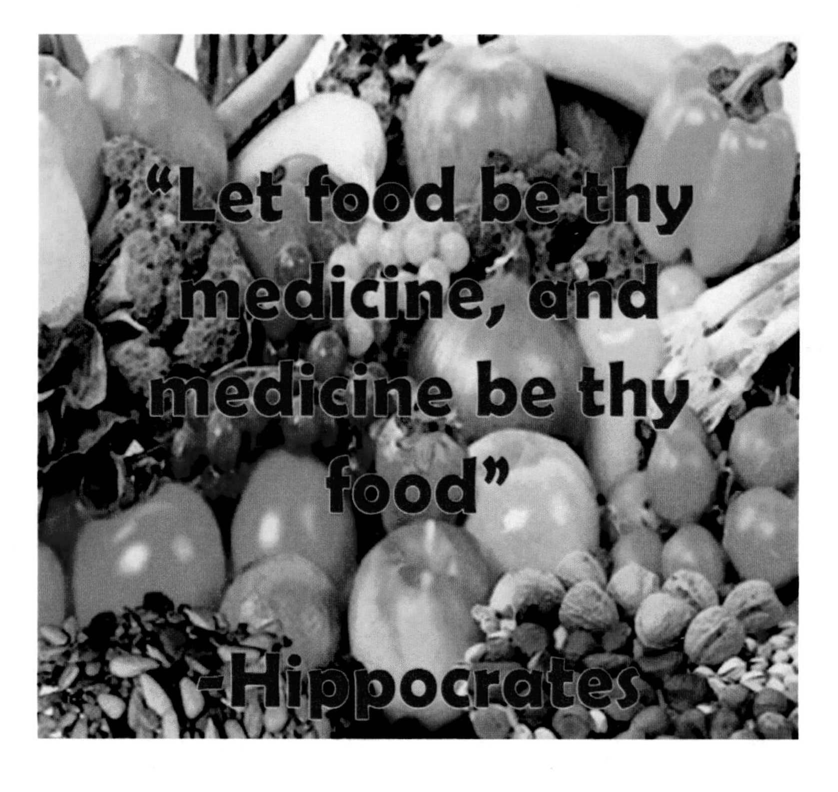

Disclaimer: Always seek the advice of your physician or other qualified health provider with any questions about your medical condition. This information is not intended to be a substitute for professional medical advice, diagnosis or treatment.

What is inflammation?

Inflammation is the body's way of mobilizing it's troops to help heal an injury. Often along with inflammation comes swelling from fluid moving to the site too. Inflammation is a good thing for acute, short-term injuries like a twisted ankle, broken bones, bug bites, or bacterial infection. In the short-term the inflammation gets your body's immune system and other healing cytokines and cellular building blocks to the scene to repair, wall off and treat the injury or infection.

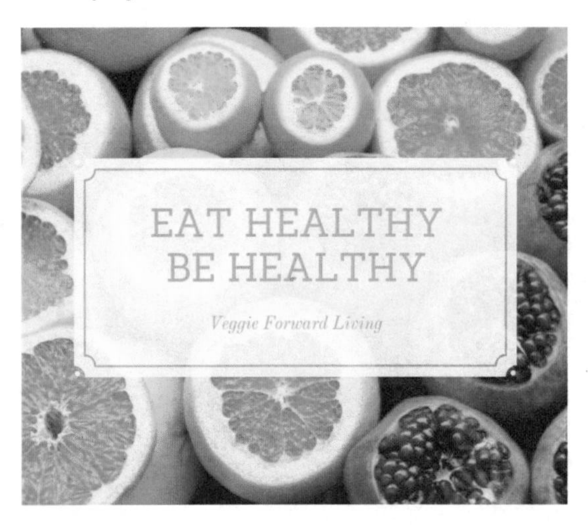

Inflammation becomes an issue when it goes on and on and on for a long period of time and there really isn't an injury (auto-immune issues) or we keep reintroducing the offending agent to our system (sugar, processed foods, etc). This is when it becomes chronic and causes pain and a dis-ease in the body. There are many studies linking high inflammation to the cause of cancers and diseases such as diabetes, high blood pressure, and pain disorders.

One of the most common causes of inflammation in most humans is bad bacteria in their GI track. It is called "bad bacteria" because it eats sugars and animal fats and other chemicals found in processed foods and then it poops and pees out things in our GI track that increase the inflammation in our bodies. That's right, these inflammation chemicals don't just stay in your intestines, they travel to all parts of your body and cause pain and mischief. So, the best way to battle these bad bacteria are to get some good bacteria. They are called good bacteria because when they eat a variety of fresh fruits and vegetables they poop and pee out chemicals that kill the bad bacteria (and also vitamins that we need to stay healthy). Viola! That is some easy battling. Feed the good guys that kill off the bad guys. That's why I invented Veggie Bingo. Studies showed that the magic number of fresh fruits and vegetables to eat is 25 in a week to decrease your body's overall inflammation. That is a lot of variety and also a pretty good quantity of plants to feed your good bacteria.

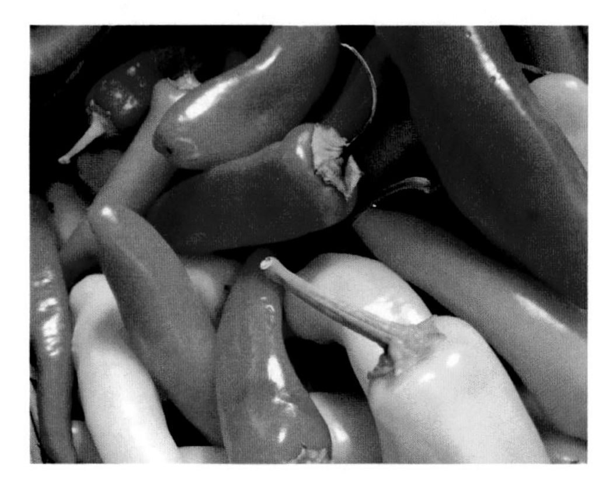

©2018 ifonfolio.com

Other great benefits of playing Veggie Bingo is that then you also don't have as much room to eat a lot of animal products. Not all fat is made equal and unfortunately animal fat is made of a higher amount of omega-6 fats. The omega-6 fats are pro-inflammatory, that means they actually cause inflammation all on their own. Our body sees those omega-6 fat molecules and sends out the troops! So that means more pain and more dis-ease in our body. When the body is in dis-ease, constantly fighting battles day in and day out, that actually leads to chronic dis-ease, which can show up as high blood pressure, increasing weight, elevated bad cholesterol (LDL), elevated blood sugar (leading to diabetes), and many others.

Inflammation doesn't just come from what we eat though. It can be caused by chemicals in our environment that we come into contact with and also can be caused by our thoughts. If you are stressed or anxious or depressed, your inflammatory chemicals in your body are higher than someone who isn't. Often your doctor will measure your cortisol level and that tells them if you have a high level of inflammation. Cortisol goes up when we are stressed or in a fight-or-flight situation and can cause trouble if it is elevated chronically. (See that list of dis-eases above.)

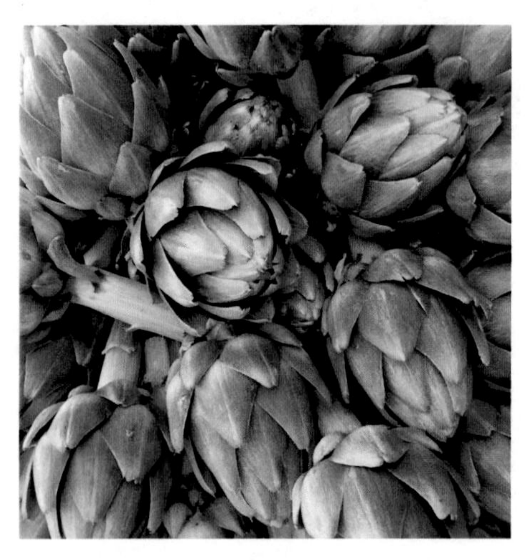

©2018 ifonfolio.com

Are there ways to battle inflammation?

Yes. Many. It helps to think of the causes and then get your battle plan ready from there. If we focus just on the inflammatory items we eat, then we just work to eliminate those items. For many of us, animal fat (especially omega 6 fats) are pro-inflammatory (cause inflammation), gluten, sugar, processed food chemicals, and to some extent night shades and animal protein. So just stop eating all of that. Yeah, right. That's pretty hard. There are inflammation battling fad diets that have you do this, but I don't recommend those as they are hard to stick to and will leave you with some nutritional holes and a whole lotta cravings. So perhaps limit those pro-inflammatory items. And add foods that have anti-inflammatory and anti-oxidant powers (omega-3 rich foods, blueberries, pineapple, eggs, walnuts, green leafy veggies, and so many more!). This includes eating a wide variety of fruits and vegetables and really having more plants than animals in your diet. We call this eating Veggie Forward in our house. Other ways to eat veggie forward in a whole and healthy way are to be vegetarian or vegan. For some people this works great, but for others it is a struggle and you may still feel hungry. So, I recommend that we all switch to the Mediterranean Lifestyle and play Veggie Bingo for decreased inflammation and greater vitality! (You can do the Mediterranean Lifestyle sans animal protein or animal products and still win the inflammation battle.)

As we've talked about, animal fat can be pro-inflammatory so if you are carrying too much of your own fat, that can actually cause you to have more pain and more inflammation. Talk about a terrible cycle! Fad diets and extreme exercise are never successful over the long-term so it is best to come up with a sustainable exercise and movement routine that works for you every day, every month, every year. Talk with your healthcare provider and see what is best for you. The goal for most of us is a calorie deficit of 150-200 calories per day. That isn't very much, but we're talking long-term here. Over time the fat comes off, the inflammation goes down, pain decreases and your vitality and health improve. I love this smaller calorie deficit because then it doesn't activate those gremlins in your brain that say "Eat ICE CREAM, Eat cookies, Get that soda!" etc. Also by adding movement to your day throughout the day and having your 45-90 minutes of exercise per day, you'll easily burn, release, and be free of the fat. Check out my online clinic for some great videos for adding movement as well as exercise: **takechargeofmyhealth.online.**

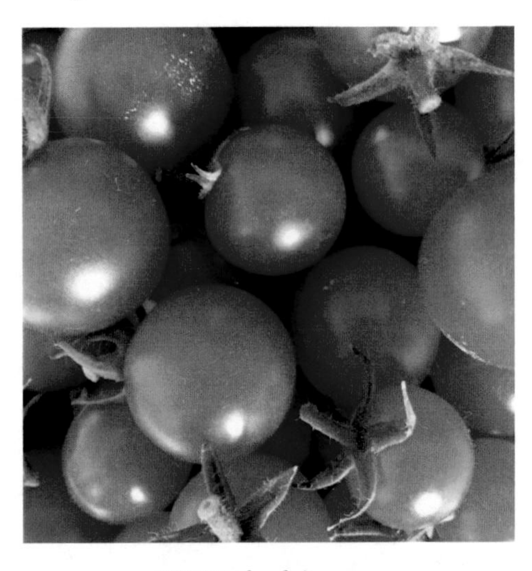

©2018 ifonfolio.com

But what we eat isn't the only thing that is increasing our inflammation, like we talked about earlier, there are a few more things you can control. We need to think about environmental toxins - what are you drinking in your water? What are you cleaning your house with? How many pesticides are on your flowers? Are you around cigarette or marijuana smoke? All these environmental things have an impact on your inflammation too. Try to eliminate or avoid as much as possible these chemicals. The single greatest impact you can make on your health is to quit smoking if you do.

The final culprit of chronic inflammation and dis-ease in our bodies is STRESS! What are your thoughts and reactions and lifestyle doing to you? Your thoughts matter. Be kind to yourself and your stress will come down. Learn to respond to situations instead of react, and your stress will come down. Can you have a less stressful lifestyle? These are the battle plans for decreasing inflammation! Love yourself and treat yourself as you would your very best friend and watch that stress melt away. Have you tried meditation, or massage, or fascial stretch therapy, or acupuncture, or walking amongst the trees, or hugging your pet, or laughing? There are so many ways to release stress from our lives. And they all feel good!

I'd be remiss as a pharmacist however if I didn't at least mention the medications called NSAIDs. That stands for Non-Steroidal Anti-inflammatory Drugs and includes such things as Advil or Ibuprofen and Aleve or naproxen. There are also prescription strength NSAIDs that your doctor would prescribe if needed. These are great for treating the acute inflammation of pain or injury but taken long term they can cause a great deal of trouble for your health and wellbeing especially impacting your stomach, intestines and kidneys. So, take them if you need them in the short term, but for long term inflammation fighting it is best to look at the root cause. What are you letting in through your nutrition, environment and thoughts?

What is the Mediterranean Lifestyle?

In one word: Awesome. Easy. Delicious. I FEEL GREAT!!! Ok that is more than one word, but you get the gist. Bruce and I were so happy to make the switch from the traditional American lifestyle to this Veggie Forward living. We both have noticed our weights decreasing, our cholesterol decreasing, our thinking improving, our sleep improving, and our energy level increasing.

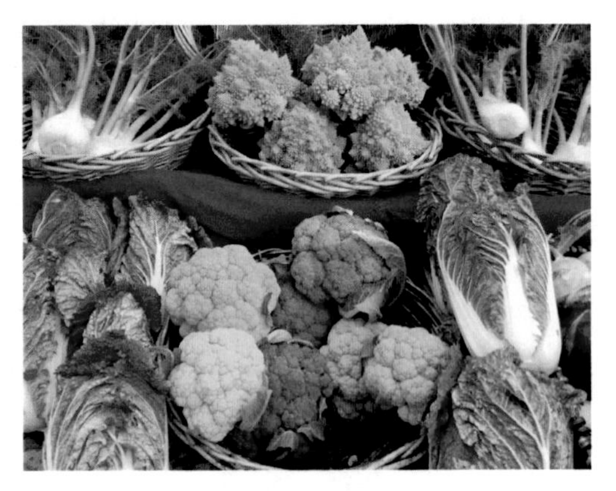

©2018 ifonfolio.com

One of the reasons weight loss, health improvements, inflammation busting, etc is so successful with the Mediterranean diet or lifestyle is that it is easy to follow and stick to. The Mediterranean Lifestyle has been studied for over 50 years because of the reported benefits for improving health and reducing overall mortality. These great results are not just from the diet consumed but the overall lifestyle that people enjoy. There is a balance between work and leisure; movement and relaxation; solitary and social time; and fresh food and convenient food products. Most important it is about enjoying life to the fullest, which includes maintaining good physical, emotional, and mental health throughout life. This is my dream for you!

The traditional Mediterranean diet and lifestyle are widely considered the gold standard for maintaining health and preventing disease. Having time to yourself is essential for mental well-being, but also having time with others to talk and laugh and go over the day's events is essential to all our lives. It is uncertain which particular component is most responsible for the positive effects of the Mediterranean Lifestyle. I think it is a combination of the healthy fresh whole foods, an active lifestyle, following traditional rather than modern labor-saving practices, and also the stress-free aspects of unplugging and not working every waking moment.

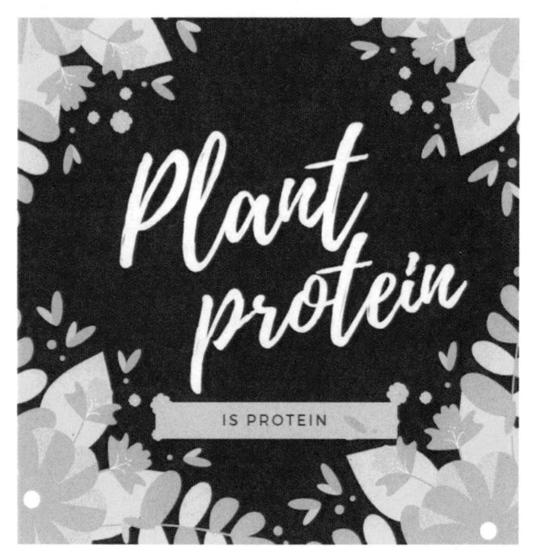

In general, the Mediterranean Lifestyle is eating a diet that is plant based, full of olive oil, nuts and fish. There is a reduced intake of animal products. As we've talked about, animal fat is highly inflammatory (and to a lesser extent so is animal protein). Humans have plenty of animal fat to begin with (at least I do!), seeing as we are animals, so to eat animal products for the majority of your caloric needs will tip the inflammation scale and lead to disease and pain. In this lifestyle, you get to choose foods that are fresh, seasonal and whole rather than processed or refined. Use simple food preparation methods, liberally using herbs, garlic and onions. Include wine with one or two meals a day and linger over the dining experiences shared with family and friends. Also, engage in regular physical activity as a part of a work or leisure. Here is the Mediterranean Lifestyle in pyramid-form.

Weekly
Sweets ≤ 2s
Potatoes ≤ 3s
Red meat < 2s
Processed meat ≤ 1s
White meat 2s
Fish/Seafood ≥ 2s
Eggs 2-4s
Legumes ≥ 2s
Every day
Dairy 2s
(preferably low fat)
Olives / Nuts / Seeds 1-2s
Herbs / Spices / Garlic / Onions
(less added salt)
Variety of flavours
Every Main Meal
Fruits 1-2 | Vegetables ≥ 2s
Variety of colours / textures
(Cooked / Raw)
Olive Oil
Bread / Pasta / Rice / Couscous/
Other cereals 1-2s
(preferably whole grain)
Water and herbal infusions
Regular physical activity
Adequate rest
Conviviality
Biodiversity and seasonality
Traditional, local
and eco-friendly products
Culinary activities
2010 edition
s = Serving

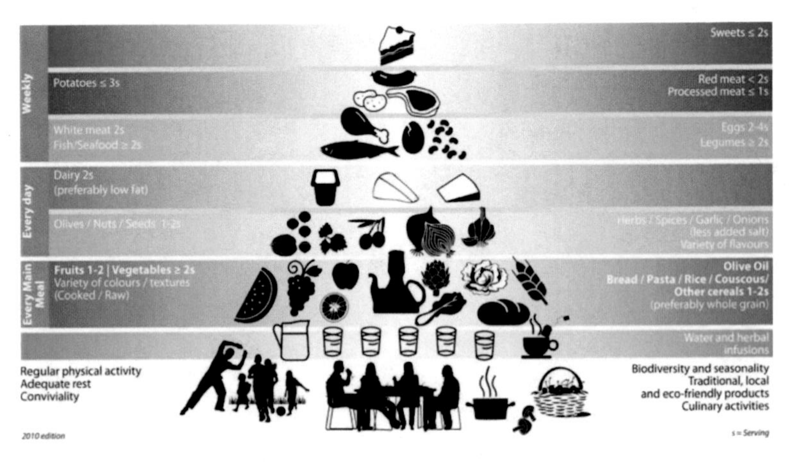

http://www.olivenews.gr/files/Mediterranean%20diet%20 Pyramid.jpg

What the studies show

This is a very truncated view of the studies, but gives you the highlights. In general, the studies have shown that adherence to the Mediterranean diet and lifestyle is inversely associated with the incidence of fatal and non-fatal heart disease, stroke, metabolic syndrome, obesity, diabetes and cancer. That's pretty powerful!

- The Seven Countries Study–overall, heart disease was rare in countries with diets that emphasized eating vegetables, whole grains, fruit, beans, fish and plant oils (Greece, Japan and Southern Italy). Also, it showed that there is a direct association between heart disease and animal fat and animal protein. Calories from refined carbohydrates (sugars) were most highly associated with non-heart mortality–that means cause of deaths not from heart attacks.

- The Lyon Diet Heart Study–there is a 50-70% reduction in risk of complications after a first heart attack if the individual switched to a Mediterranean diet. Also, this study found there might also be protection from cancer. (So it's never too late to start living this way!)

- GSSI Study–the risk of death was three times lower in patients who already had cardiovascular disease who followed the Mediterranean diet compared to a Western diet. (Again, what are we waiting for, it's never too late!)

- MORGEN Study–a diet rich in ALA (omega-3 fatty acids derived from plants) is protective against strokes.

- A meta-analysis and systematic review published in 2009 by Banel showed that walnut-supplemented diets resulted in a significant reduction in total and LDL (bad) cholesterol due to their antioxidant and anti-inflammatory effects.

- OmniHeart Trial–Mediterranean diet was more effective than either a high-carbohydrate or a high-protein diet in improving insulin sensitivity. Sticking with the

Mediterranean lifestyle is associated with 19% reduction in the risk of type 2 diabetes.

- Northern Manhattan Study – Mediterranean diet may be protective against stroke.
- PREDIMED Study—28.2% of participants who had metabolic syndrome (high blood pressure, high cholesterol, overweight) at baseline experienced a reversal of the syndrome while on the Mediterranean diet compared to those who followed a low-fat diet.

So that is pretty compelling that not only do you win the battle of inflammation, you can totally increase your *healthspan*! The goal in this life isn't to just live a long time (lifespan) but to do so healthfully and independently and with some joy. That's your *healthspan*. And isn't it so great that you can do it so easily by eating delicious foods and simply playing Veggie Bingo!

The food

Olive oil is one of the most eaten food items in the Mediterranean diet. This omega-9 fat has many beneficial effects including: improvements in blood pressure, plasma glucose, insulin sensitivity, total cholesterol/HDL (good cholesterol) ratio, and endothelial function. Other good sources of fats in the Mediterranean diet include olives, avocados, nut butter, nuts and seeds.

There is a great deal of dietary diversity as well. This means that you eat a wide variety of whole foods, especially focusing on what is in season in your area. I encourage you to play Veggie Bingo© weekly to help ensure you are getting a large variety of foods. The more diverse fruits and vegetables you eat, the better the health of the good bacteria in your GI tract. The more good bacteria you have then the less bad bacteria. Less bad bacteria leads to less total-body inflammation and pain. So enjoy Veggie Bingo© and feeling great!

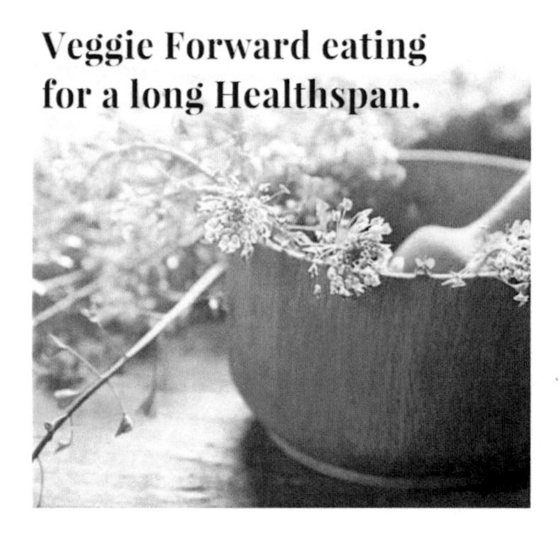

One of the most powerful impacts on health comes from adopting an attitude of leisurely enjoyment of meals. Let eating food be pleasurable! Not pictured, is the tradition of having wine with dinner. Recommended is to drink 1-2 glasses of wine daily or per social convention. There are a lot of studies coming out about alcohol, but in general women are to have 1 glass a day (or 7 glasses/week) and men 1-2 glasses a day (or 7-14 glasses/week). More alcohol than these guidelines greatly increases the risks of all cancer. England has already adopted these new recommendations. If you are interested in more about alcohol check out the Netflix documentary, *The Truth About Alcohol*.

The basics guidelines for the food are:

1. Vegetables - the more the merrier!
2. Legumes–beans instead of bread
3. Fruit–the perfect dessert!

4. Nuts–eat a healthy handful everyday, and when in doubt walnuts
5. Fish–more fish, less meat
6. Olive Oil–all the time!
7. Dairy–if you eat it, make it low fat or non-fat, and not too much
8. Alcohol–a little goes a long way, red over white, wine over all else

Making the Switch to the Mediterranean Lifestyle

Any big change in diet or nutrition can be daunting, so to make it easier think about just a step-by-step approach. Here are some simple suggestions of new options to add to your life to help you convert to the Mediterranean Lifestyle:

- Replace 1 or 2 meat meals each week with fish to change the composition of fat consumed. More omega 3's and less omega 6's to continue reducing inflammation.
- Playing Veggie Bingo adds more daily servings of vegetables in a fun way.
- Eat the rainbow! Emphasizing more colorful fruits and vegetables will increase the amount of antioxidants you intake. Again battling that inflammation with every bite!
- Substitute fresh fruit for one dessert per week. Even if you don't usually eat dessert, plan a weekly meal that begins or ends in fresh fruit will be a helpful dietary change.

- Switch from refined bread and grains to whole grain products.
- Substitute beans for grains a couple times a week. (Remember: hummus is beans and olive oil, that makes for an easy meal with fresh veggies)
- Get in the nut habit–have them handy for snacks.
- Switch cocktails for antioxidant and anti-inflammatory-rich wine. Red has more antioxidant power, but white wine has some too.
- Dip whole wheat bread into olive oil & herbs instead of butter.
- Use avocado on sandwiches instead of mayonnaise.
- Order fish instead of meat when out (grilled or sautéed in olive oil).
- Add nuts to salads instead of cheese.
- Make it a habit to cook with cold-pressed organic extra virgin olive oil. The smoke point is lower than other oils so be careful not to over heat the pan. I set off the smoke detector at least once a month when I'm too excited about eating and get the pan too hot. D'Oh!
- Use mushrooms instead of meat in typical meat-based sauces or dishes.
- Switch to 1% or fat-free milk (and eventually switch completely to sugar-free organic almond milk).
- Use more herbs and spices to cut back on salt when cooking.

- If you need a quick snack, Kind® bars are great options (just check the sugar content before you buy).
- Give going vegan a try. Make 3 meals a week vegan to really fight inflammation. Completely switching to a vegan lifestyle can be too daunting and stressful for many people which then makes it hard to stick with, but 3 meals a week is totally do-able.

How Much To Eat

Your body has come with easy measuring devices for your nutrition needs: your hands! A tightly cupped hand is great for measuring fats and seeds. A lightly cupped hand measures nuts, whole grains and protein. And two open hands measures fruit and vegetable servings for your meal. Typically, I use one handful for each fruit or veggie I'm adding to a recipe or meal. For example, when time is tight in the morning I make my Favorite Breakfast Shake and add in 1 handful of walnuts for me, then 1 handful of walnuts for Bruce, 1 handful of blueberries for me, 1 handful of blueberries for Bruce, etc. That way the shake makes a great meal and even proportions for the both of us. This may be more challenging if your spouse is much bigger than you, so use your best judgement. You've got this!

The Japanese practice something that my clients and I love and I hope you will too. It's called "hara hachi bu". You say the phrase out loud before eating and then stop when you figure you are 80% full. Specifically, this practice of mindful eating is performed by the Okinawan people. The eating practices of the Okinawans came under research because they have a large population, mostly men, that live to be 100 years old. Of course, it helps to eat healthy food as well, but simply learning to eat until you are 80% full would do wonders for everyone. It is also an easy way to create a 150-200 calorie deficit, so if you are trying to lose a few pounds, over the course of a month you'll drop 2 pounds safely and easily. One of my clients loves this so much she had a sign made for her dining room table so they always remember *hara hachi bu*!

Eat real food.
Not too much.
Mostly plants.
-Michael Polla

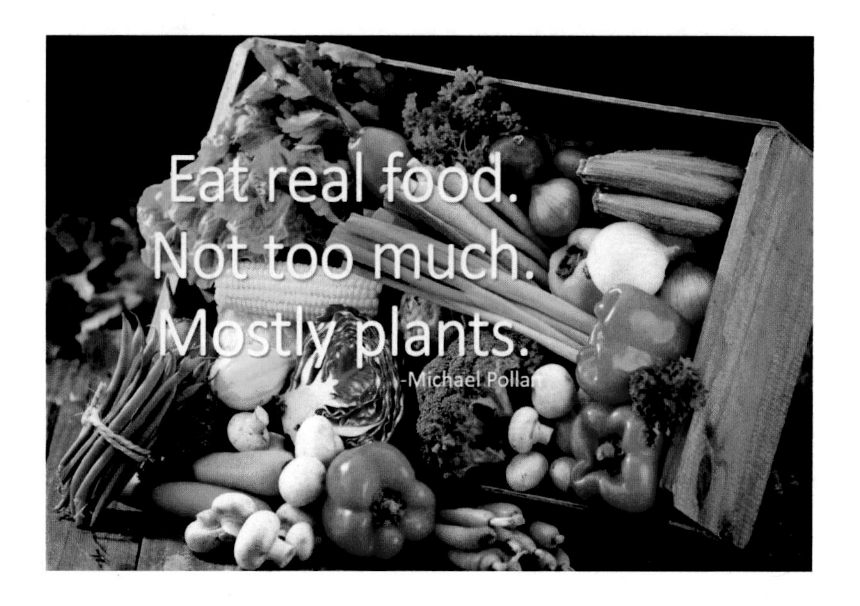

What are the health impacts of Veggie Forward Mediterranean Lifestyle living?

1. Decrease total body inflammation.
2. Decrease pain.
3. Decrease blood pressure.
4. Decrease risk of cancer.
5. Decrease bad (LDL) cholesterol.

6. Decrease blood sugar/Maintain healthy blood sugar.
7. Decrease weight/Maintain healthy weight.
8. Live longer.

In the Adventist Health Study, a 30 year old vegetarian man will live 9.5 years longer than the average Californian 30 year old man. And a 30 year old vegetarian woman will live 6.1 years longer than the average Californian 30 year old woman.

The "superfoods" in a mostly vegetarian diet that have an especially strong impact on health and longevity were listed in the December 2003 Nutrition Action Health Letter and included: sweet potatoes, grape tomatoes, fat-free or 1% milk, broccoli, salmon, whole grain crackers, brown rice, citrus fruits, butternut squash, and greens including kale and spinach. Foods also consumed in abundance by 100 year-olds include nuts, blueberries, olive oil, avocados, bell peppers, soybeans, flaxseed, Brussel sprouts, legumes, apples, red wine, coffee, tea, vegetable juices and whole grains.

How to Play Veggie Bingo

- This book contains 1 years' worth of Veggie Bingo cards. (And some really fun bad jokes.)
- The goal is to eat one serving of each fruit or vegetable listed on the bingo card in a week. Mark off the fruit or vegetable after you've eaten a serving. Your goal is a blackout bingo card each week!
- For most foods, a serving size is a handful. Use your own hand size as a judge for what your body needs.

Bananas can be tricky and often ½ of a banana is a serving.

- I recommend starting a new card on Sundays - or whenever you do your grocery shopping.
- Take your card with you to the grocery store to make shopping easier.
- Veggie forward recipes are included for you to give you some ideas.
- Have fun, fight inflammation, and feel better!

Onward to Veggie Bingo!

Get ready for a fun way to feel better, eat better and have more vitality. I've arranged the Veggie Bingo cards in order of seasons and included some recipes as examples of ways to eat Veggie Forward. Food is so much a part of the global market now and you can get almost anything in any season. But some things are going to be easier to get in the winter than in the summer and vice versa. So I've tried to make things easier for when you are going to the store or out to eat. You can cut the cards out of the book and put them on your refrigerator or kitchen counter for the week to stay engaged. One of my client couples has weekly wagers for who not only gets the Veggie Bingo, but who gets it first! My favorite was their wager that the winner got to sleep in on the weekend and the non-winner was on puppy duty.

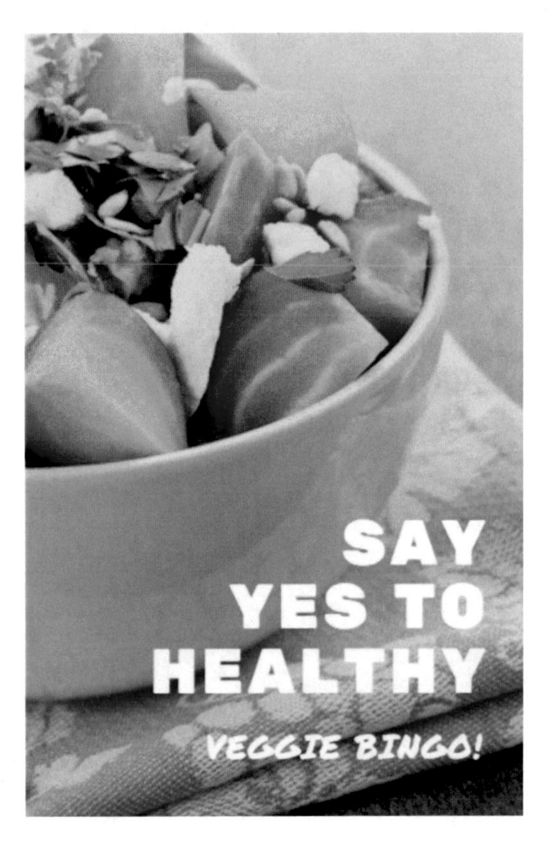

You'll also find that some of these veggies, God help ya, you just don't like. That's ok, substitute it for another whole fresh fruit or veggie that you do like. For example, you'll notice there are not a lot of eggplant, beets, or brussels sprouts on these cards. That's because Bruce and I don't like them. So feel free to put them in your card if you do.

My favorite Veggie Forward cookbook for eating at home and throwing parties is: Love Real Food by Kathryne Taylor.

Ways to make winning Veggie Bingo easier are to go to Veggie Forward restaurants and grocery stores that do the prep-work and cooking for you. I'm all for cooking at home, but some days are just too busy. We love to go to New Seasons, Market of

Choice and Whole Foods for their deli and hot wok items. They have done the chopping and cooking and we just get to eat the Veggie Forward deliciousness at a pretty reasonable price. Trader Joes also has great organic options already chopped and ready for you to throw in the skillet for quick lunches and dinners. Many restaurants are making the switch to Veggie Forward living so keep your eyes and ears open. Here in the Portland, Oregon area we like Laughing Planet, Lucky Lab Brewery, Andina, and Gabagool.

I hope you enjoy your Veggie Bingo and get a chuckle out of the jokes.

Happy Eating! Happy Living!

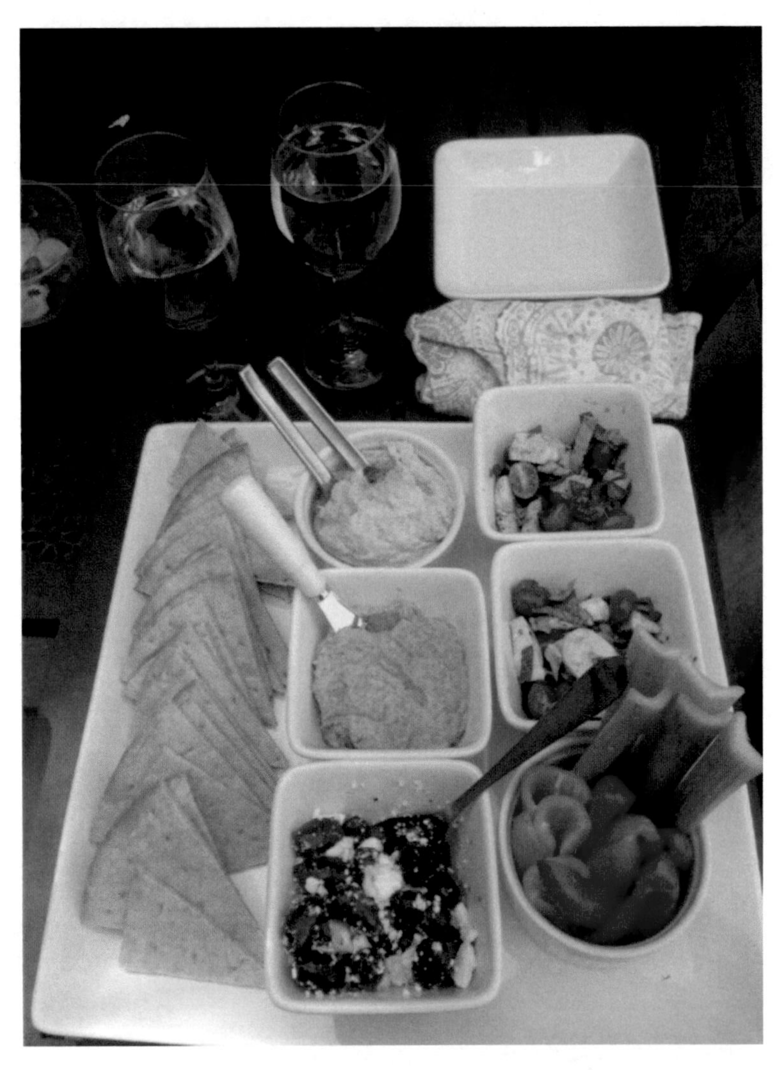

An example of a veggie forward, Mediterranean Lifestyle dinner. Whole wheat pita, hummus, green goddess avocado dip, feta and kalamata olives, and a caprese salad. Delish!

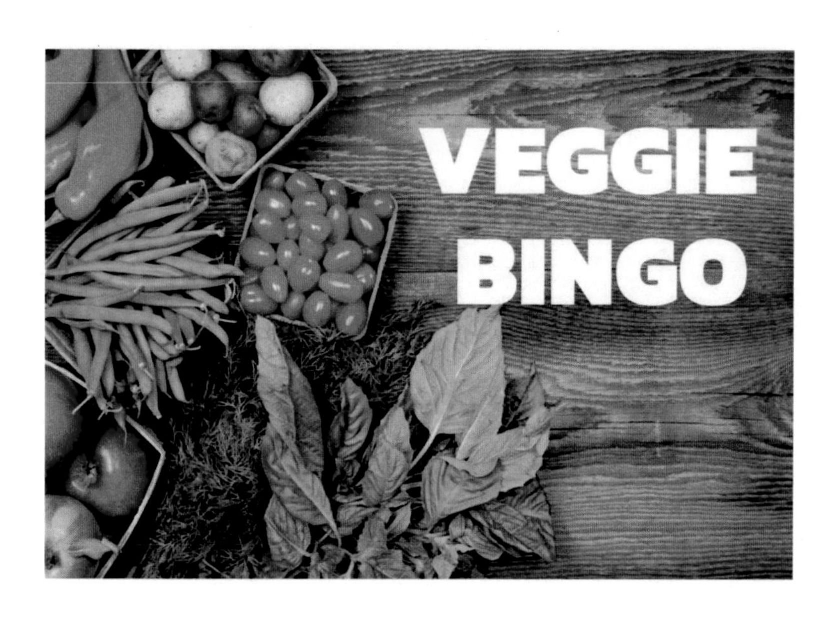
VEGGIE
BINGO

V	E	GG	I	E
Mango	Avocado	Jalapeño	Green Beans	Cauliflower
Spinach	Red Leaf Lettuce	Green Onion	Purple Onion	Tomato
Yellow Pepper	Zucchini	You Choose ________	Lemons	Broccolini
Carrots	Parsnip	Asparagus	Bananas	Orange (or cutie)
Kale	Bok Choy	Blueberries	Pineapple	Corn

Do not eat items you have an allergy to. Substitute with a different healthy whole fruit or vegetable of your choice.

Winter Week 1

V	E	GG	I	E
Banana	Avocado	Green Pepper	Green Beans	Strawberry
Corn	Apple	Broccoflower (Romanesco)	Purple Onion	Tomato
Yellow Pepper	Zucchini	You Choose ________	Lemons	Broccolini
Carrots	Red Pepper	Cucumber	Olives	Orange (or cutie)
Kale	Bok Choy	Blueberries	Pineapple	Spinach

Do not eat items you have an allergy to. Substitute with a different healthy whole fruit or vegetable of your choice.

Winter Week 2

What do you use to open a banana?

A Monkey!

Avgolemono Soup

Ingredients

8 cups chicken stock (or vegetable stock)

1 cup cooked chicken, shredded

1 cup orzo pasta

1 medium white onion - chopped

4 carrots, chopped

4 stalks celery, chopped

½ teaspoon oregano

Salt & Pepper to taste

2 eggs

2 lemons, juiced

Handful of fresh dill, chopped

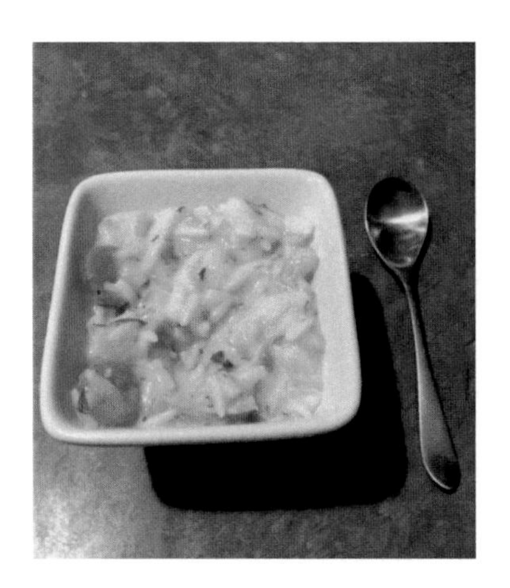

MAKES 6 SERVINGS

In large stock pot, place the chicken stock, chicken, orzo, onion, carrots, celery, oregano, salt and pepper.

Bring to a boil and simmer until vegetables are tender and orzo is cooked (~10-12 minutes).

Remove pot from heat.

Whisk eggs in separate bowl until frothy. Add in lemon juice and continue to whisk. Slowly whisk in some of the liquid from the hot soup to temper the eggs. Do this 3-4 times so the eggs will not congeal. Then mix the egg sauce into the soup. Stir in the fresh dill and serve.

Enjoy!

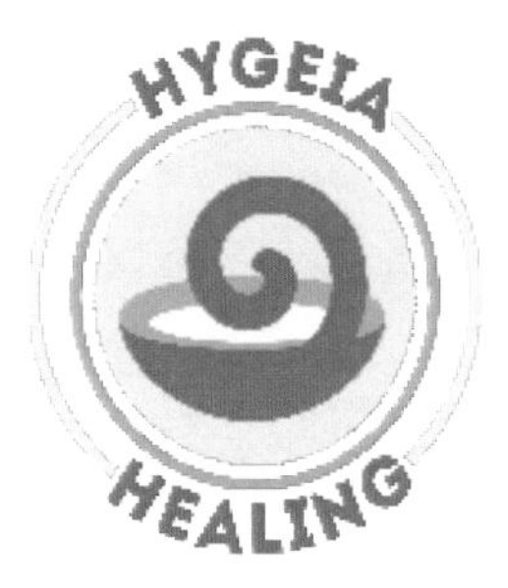

V	E	GG	I	E
Fennel	Avocado	Green Pepper	Yellow squash	Lemon
Corn	Banana	Cabbage	Purple Onion	Tomato
Kale	Zucchini	You Choose ________	Mushroom	Broccoli
Carrots	Red Pepper	Cucumber	Radish	Grapefruit
Celery	Bok Choy	Blueberries	Romaine lettuce	Spinach

Do not eat items you have an allergy to. Substitute with a different healthy whole fruit or vegetable of your choice.

Winter Week 3

Dori's Tortellini soup

Ingredients

8 cups chicken stock

1 pound mild Italian sausage

1 bag (2-3 cups) fresh baby spinach

1 28oz can Italian Stewed tomatoes

9 oz. bag of pesto tortellini (can find at Trader Joes)

Parmesan cheese to garnish

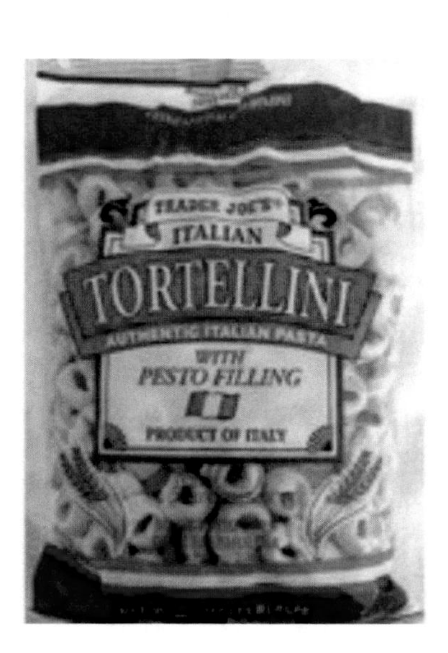

COOKING

In large stock pot, cook the mild Italian sausage until browned. Remove and set aside. Drain fat.

In the large stock pot bring the chicken stock to a slow boil. Add in spinach, tomatoes and the already cooked sausage. Add in the tortellini and cook according to directions (usually 7-12 minutes depending on the brand). Once tortellini are tender, ladle into bowls and garnish with cheese.

Total cooking time 30-40 minutes.

Enjoy!

Many thanks to Dori Hamilton for this great recipe.

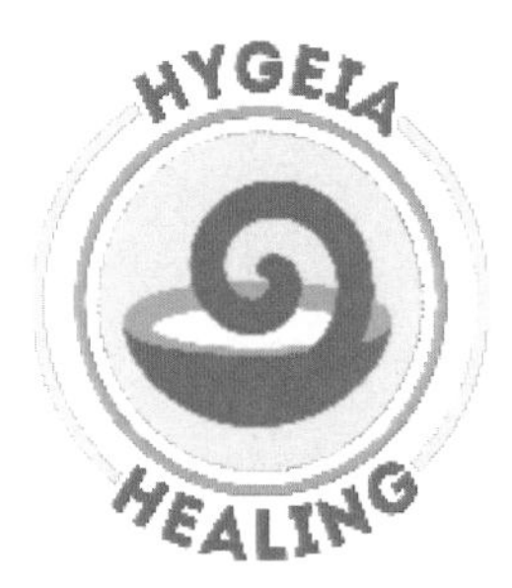

V	E	GG	I	E
grapes	broccolini	Green Pepper	Yellow squash	kale
Corn	banana	apple	onion	Tomato
Green beans	Zucchini	You Choose ________	mushroom	avocado
Carrots	Red Pepper	Cucumber	Brussel sprouts	Strawberry
celery	peas	Blueberries	Butter lettuce	Spinach

Do not eat items you have an allergy to. Substitute with a different healthy whole fruit or vegetable of your choice.

Winter Week 4

V	E	GG	I	E
Celery	White Onion	Purple Onion	Green Chilies	Corn
Carrots	Red Potato	Red bell pepper	Green Bell Pepper	Oranges
Tomatoes	Green Beans	You Choose ________	Olives	Zucchini
Broccoli	Spinach	Cranberries	Banana	Apples
Pumpkin	Mushrooms	Cilantro*	Pear	Brussel sprouts

Do not eat items you have an allergy to. Substitute with a different healthy whole fruit or vegetable of your choice.

** Fresh cilantro may not technically be considered a veggie However it is a green leafy item that is great for cleaning out The GI tract and the liver.*

Winter Week 5

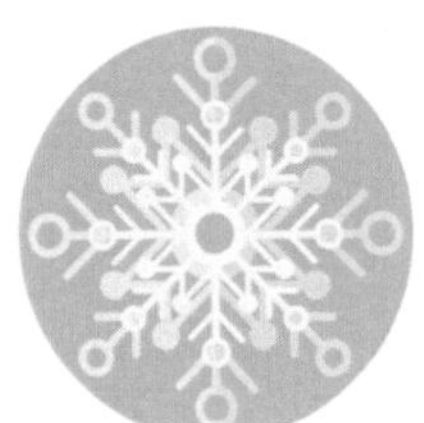

Why did the chicken get kicked out of school?

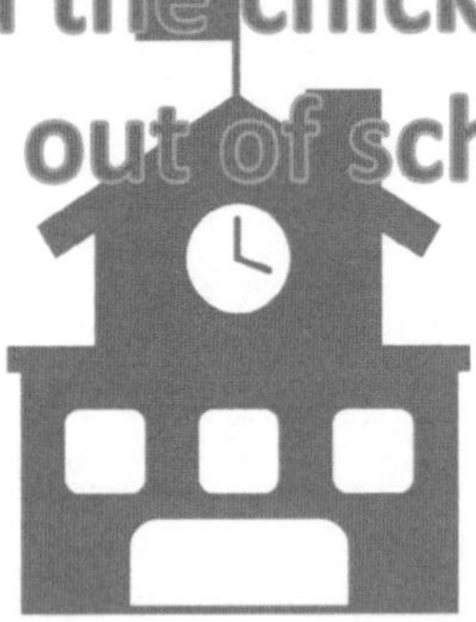

Because of his fowl language!

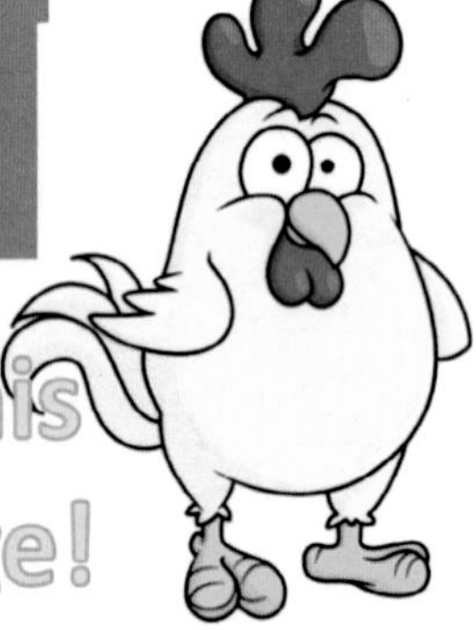

V	E	GG	I	E
Grapes	Broccoli	Green Pepper	Cilantro or Parsley *	Jalapeño
Cauliflower	Banana	Apple	Onion	Tomato
Green beans	Zucchini	You Choose ________	Mushroom	Parsnip
Rainbow Carrots	Yellow Pepper	Cucumber	Beet	Brussels Sprouts
Orange or cutie	Peas	Blueberries	Sweet Potato	Spinach

Do not eat items you have an allergy to. Substitute with a different healthy whole fruit or vegetable of your choice.

** Fresh cilantro or parsley may not technically be considered a veggie However they are green leafy items that are great for cleaning out The GI tract and the liver.*

Winter Week 6

V	E	GG	I	E
Cabbage	Red bell pepper	Serrano pepper	Cilantro*	Grapefruit
Carrot	Yellow Onion	Avocado	Bok choy	Banana
Cranberries	Green beans	You Choose ________	Zucchini	Lemon
Broccoli	Arugula	Apricot	Mushrooms	Beets
Potato	Tomato	Red onion	Olives	Red Leaf Lettuce

Do not eat items you have an allergy to. Substitute with a different healthy whole fruit or vegetable of your choice.

*** Fresh cilantro may not technically be considered a veggie However it is a green leafy item that is great for cleaning out The GI tract and the liver.*

Winter Week 7

V	E	GG	I	E
Peas	Apple	Banana	Blueberries	Strawberry
Cabbage	Yellow onion	Avocado	Bok choy	Orange
Cranberries	Green beans	You Choose ________	Zucchini	Olives
Broccoli	Lettuce	Leek	Mushrooms	Parsley*
Red Potato	Cauliflower	Persimmon	Olives	Butternut squash

Do not eat items you have an allergy to. Substitute with a different healthy whole fruit or vegetable of your choice.
** Fresh parsley may not technically be considered a veggie*
However it is a green leafy item that is great for cleaning out
The GI tract and the liver.

Winter Week 8

Sunshine Pasta

Ingredients

1 pound mild Italian sausage

1 purple onion - chopped into big pieces

2 cups/heads broccolini - chopped

1 cup sliced cherry tomatoes

Juice of 2 lemons

Fresh rigatoni or elbow macaroni cooked per directions

Salt & Pepper to taste

COOKING

In large skillet cook the sausage until slightly caramelized. Remove from pan and set aside on plate lined with paper towels to remove excess fat.

In pan, keeping only about 1 Tablespoon of the fat, sauté the purple onion and broccolini. Once done to your likeness - we like our veggies cooked but still firm and crunchy. Turn off the heat and add in the tomatoes and lemon juice. Toss together with pasta. Salt and Pepper to taste. Serve and enjoy!

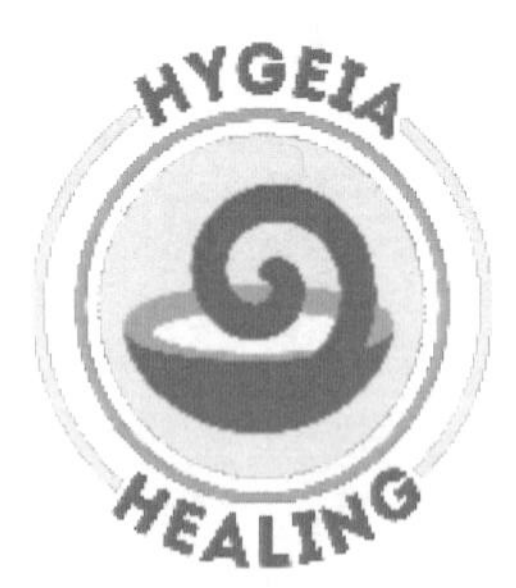

V	E	GG	I	E
Orange or cutie	Apple	Banana	Blueberries	Pineapple
Mango	Spinach	Bok Choy	Kale	Cherry tomatoes
Purple Onion	Broccolini	You Choose ________	Potato	Corn
Peas	Green Beans	Cauliflower	Red Bell Pepper	Green Chilies
Jalapeño	Zucchini	Squash of your choosing	Carrots	Celery

Do not eat items you have an allergy to. Substitute with a different healthy whole fruit or vegetable of your choice.

Winter Week 9

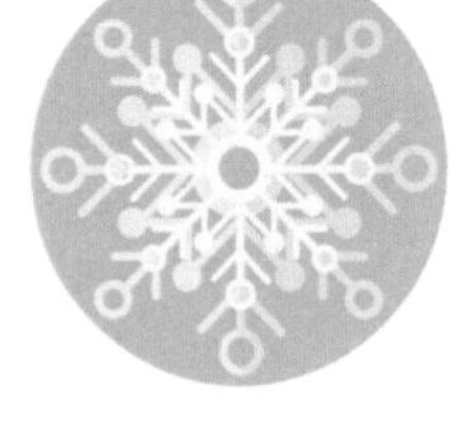

How many pastry chefs does it take to make a pie?

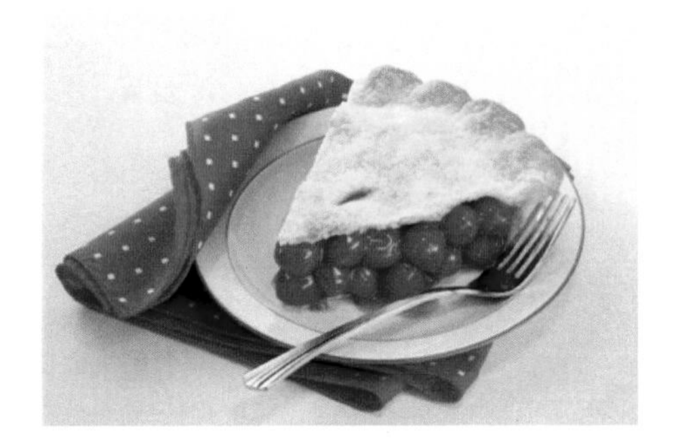

3.14

V	E	GG	I	E
Grapefruit	Apple	Green beans	Onion	Cherry Tomatoes
Broccoli	Bell Peppers	Baby Corn	Ginger*	Sweet Potato
Kale	Zucchini	You Choose ________	Mushroom	Bamboo shoots
Carrots	Cabbage	Cucumber	Bok choy	Grapefruit
Celery	Artichoke hearts	Blueberries	Olives	Spinach

Do not eat items you have an allergy to. Substitute with a different healthy whole fruit or vegetable of your choice.
** Fresh ginger may not technically be considered a veggie*
But it is fresh and delightful!

Winter Week 10

V	E	GG	I	E
Mango	Avocado	Grapefruit	Green Beans	Cauliflower
Spinach	Red Leaf Lettuce	Green Onion	Purple Onion	Tomato
Yellow Pepper	Zucchini	You Choose ________	Lemons	Broccolini
Carrots	Parsnip	Asparagus	Bananas	Orange (or cutie)
Kale	Bok Choy	Blueberries	Pineapple	Corn

Do not eat items you have an allergy to. Substitute with a different healthy whole fruit or vegetable of your choice.

Winter Week 11

V	E	GG	I	E
Black Olives	Leeks	Green Beans	Corn	Peas
Zucchini	Broccoli	Carrots	Celery	Onion
Spinach	Butter Lettuce	You Choose ________	Raspberries	Pomegranate
Cherry Tomatoes	Romaine Lettuce	Bell Pepper	Artichoke Hearts	Apple
Cucumber	Radish	Mushrooms	Banana	Butternut squash

Do not eat items you have an allergy to. Substitute with a different healthy whole fruit or vegetable of your choice.

Winter Week 12

Where do chickens grow?

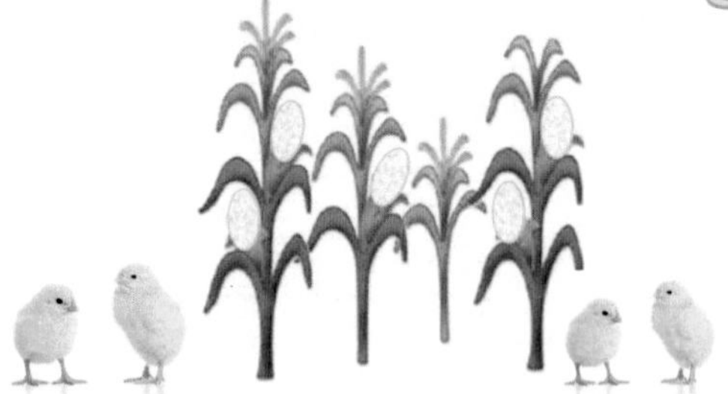

On Egg Plants!

V	E	GG	I	E
Pineapple	Snow peas	Corn	Basil*	Cherry Tomatoes
Blackberries	Grapes	Banana	Red onion	Mushrooms
Green Swish Chard	Kale	You Choose ________	Spaghetti squash	Parsley or Basil*
Kalamata Olives	Grapefruit	Mango	Peach	Bok Choy
Asparagus	Radish	Carrots	Celery	Spinach

Do not eat items you have an allergy to. Substitute with a different healthy whole fruit or vegetable of your choice.
** Fresh basil and parsley may not technically be considered veggies, However they are green leafy items that are great for cleaning out The GI tract and the liver.*

Winter Week 13

Burrito bowls

Makes 6-8 big servings

Ingredients:

Quinoa

Chicken Stock (4 cups = 1 box)

2 limes

Cilantro

Black beans (canned organic)

Corn (canned organic)

Salt & Pepper

2 T chopped garlic (buy pre-chopped in jar)

1 T olive oil

1 chopped red onion

1 chopped green bell pepper

1 chopped yellow bell pepper

1 chopped red bell pepper

1 chopped orange bell pepper

1 chopped zucchini

1 chopped yellow squash

1 can drained chopped tomatoes

1 chopped jalapeño

1 can diced green chilies

2 cups chopped roasted chicken

Chili powder and Salt & Pepper

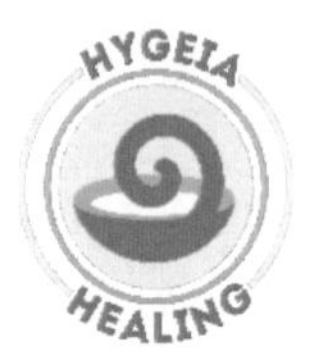

QUINOA PREPARATION

To make the quinoa, in a large pot combine 4 cups of chicken stock and 2 cups quinoa. Bring to a boil, then cover and simmer for 15 minutes (give or take a few minutes). Once the liquid is absorbed, sprinkle with ground salt and pepper to taste, stir in drained and rinsed black beans and corn. Add in the juice of 2 limes and a healthy handful of chopped cilantro.

Set aside.

BOWL PREPARATION

Put all ingredients in large pot or skillet. Cook with lid on and frequent stirring on medium heat for 10-15 minutes until veggies are cooked to your desire. Add chili powder and salt and pepper to your taste. I like it spicy so I add 1 T chili powder to the roasted chicken to coat it then add it to the pot.

Once the quinoa and veggie mixture is completed, dish out large spoonful of each into a bowl. Garnish with avocado and cheese! Viola!

This is a simple, delicious meal that is perfect for lunches and dinner during the week. Makes 6-8 hearty portions.

V	E	GG	I	E
Grapes	Broccoli	Green Pepper	Cilantro or Parsley *	Jalapeño
Cauliflower	Banana	Apple	Onion	Tomato
Green Beans	Zucchini	You Choose ________	Mushroom	Avocado
Rainbow Carrots	Yellow Pepper	Cucumber	Olives	Strawberry
Orange or cutie	Peas	Blueberries	Sweet potato	Spinach

Do not eat items you have an allergy to. Substitute with a different healthy whole fruit or vegetable of your choice.

** Fresh cilantro or parsley may not technically be considered a veggie However they are green leafy items that are great for cleaning out The GI tract and the liver.*

Spring Week 1

V	E	GG	I	E
Snow Peas	Baby Corn	Red Pepper	Green Pepper	Mushroom s
Bok choy	Onion	Carrots	Watercress	Broccoli
Spinach	Kale	You Choose ________	Romaine Lettuce	Beets
Cabbage	Celery	Strawberry	Banana	Apple
Orange	Blueberries	Basil*	Tomatoes	Radish

Do not eat items you have an allergy to. Substitute with a different healthy whole fruit or vegetable of your choice.
** Fresh Basil may not technically be considered a veggie*
However it is a green leafy item packed full of vitamins!

Spring Week 2

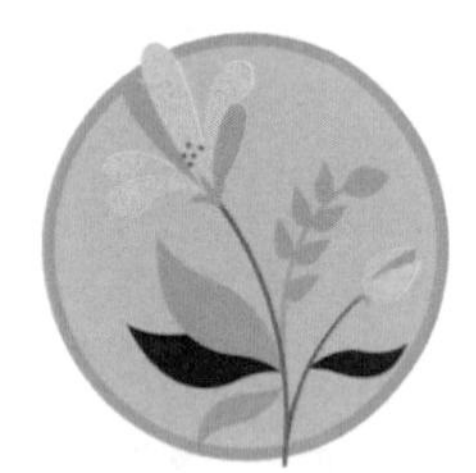

V E GG I E

Zucchini	Yellow Squash	Red Pepper	Green Pepper	Green Beans
Romaine lettuce	Purple Onion	Celery	Green Chilies	Broccoli
Spinach	Strawberries	You Choose ________	Limes	Carrots
Kiwi	Avocado	Strawberries	Banana	Apple
Grapefruit	Blueberries	Cilantro*	Tomatoes	Corn

Do not eat items you have an allergy to. Substitute with a different healthy whole fruit or vegetable of your choice.
** Fresh Cilantro may not technically be considered a veggie*
However it is a green leafy item great for cleansing and detoxing!

Spring Week 3

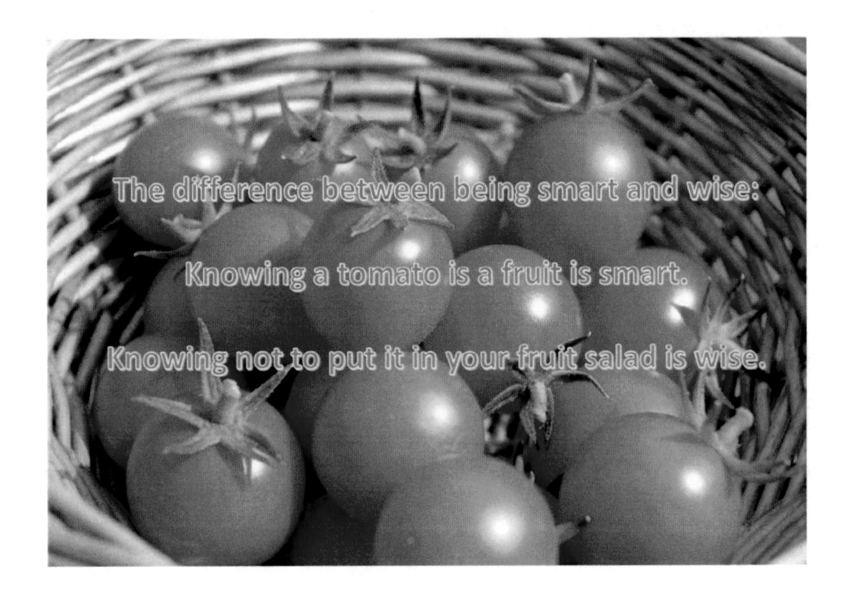
The difference between being smart and wise:
Knowing a tomato is a fruit is smart.
Knowing not to put it in your fruit salad is wise.

V	E	GG	I	E
Zucchini	Orange	Red Pepper	Green Pepper	Beets
Romaine lettuce	Purple Onion	Kalamata olives	cucumber	Broccoli
Spinach	Strawberries	You Choose ________	lemon	Celery
Pineapple	Rainbow carrots	Peaches	Banana	Apple
Mango	Blueberries	Parsley*	Jicama	Cherry Tomatoes

Do not eat items you have an allergy to. Substitute with a different healthy whole fruit or vegetable of your choice.

** Fresh Parsley may not technically be considered a veggie*
However it is a green leafy item great for cleansing and detoxing!

Spring Week 4

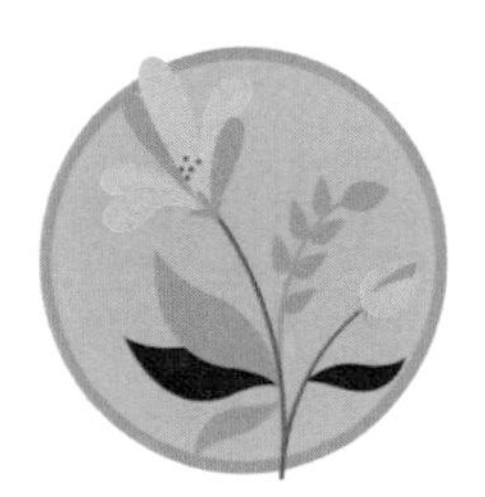

Coconut Curry

Makes 4 big servings

Ingredients:

1 can coconut milk

1 Tablespoonful turmeric powder

1 Tablespoon curry powder (or to your liking)

1 teaspoonful coriander powder

Salt & Pepper

1-2 cups chopped roasted chicken (if desired)

1-2 T olive oil

2 cloves garlic minced

Chopped Veggies I recommend:

Purple onion, green beans, red bell pepper, green bell pepper, zucchini, yellow squash, snow peas, broccoli, carrots, tomatoes

½ cup chopped cilantro

Brown rice (I cook organic brown rice in chicken stock for extra flavor, but to make this completely vegetarian omit the chicken and cook rice in vegetable broth or water.)

SAUCE PREPARATION

Mix together the coconut milk, turmeric, curry and coriander powder. This will be a beautiful bright yellow. Give it a taste and add more spices and salt and pepper to your liking. Keep in mind the veggies and rice will make it less spicy when done.

Set aside.

PUTTING IT TOGETHER

In a large skillet add olive oil and when heated add chopped veggies. Cook for ~6-10 minutes to your desired level of tenderness. Add the coconut curry sauce and heat until bubbly.

Serve over brown rice and garnish lavishly with cilantro.

Viola!

This is a simple, delicious meal that is a quick dinner as most veggies can be purchased already chopped OR chopped in advance. This meal fights inflammation because of the high turmeric amount and multiple veggies.

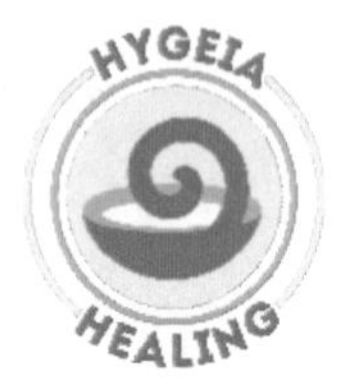

V	E	GG	I	E
Sweet Potato	Peach	Red Pepper	Grapes	Mushrooms
Celery	Green Onion	Asparagus	Olives	Edamame
Broccoli	Basil*	You Choose ________	Avocado	beets
Banana	Blueberries	Grapefruit	Zucchini	Apple
Yellow Squash	Cucumber	Orange	Peach	Tomatoes

Do not eat items you have an allergy to. Substitute with a different healthy whole fruit or vegetable of your choice.
** Fresh Basil may not technically be considered a veggie*
However it is a green leafy item packed full of vitamins!

Spring Week 5

Curried Chicken Salad

Makes 4 big servings

Ingredients:

1 cup fat-free plain Greek yogurt

1 Tablespoonful turmeric powder

2-3 teaspoonfuls curry powder (or to your liking)

1 teaspoonful coriander powder

Salt & Pepper

1-2 cups chopped roasted chicken (for vegetarian option replace with 1 can rinsed chickpeas)

1 small chopped red onion

3 chopped celery stalks

1 cup red seedless grapes sliced in half

1 cup chopped walnuts

¼ -1/2 cup chopped cilantro (to your liking)

1 -2 carrots grated

Romain lettuce if desired

Whole wheat crackers, pita, or bread

SAUCE PREPARATION

Mix together the yogurt, turmeric, curry and coriander powder. This will be a beautiful bright yellow. Give it a taste and add more spices and salt and pepper to your liking.

Set aside.

PUTTING IT TOGETHER

Mix together the yogurt sauce with the chicken, onion, celery, walnuts and grapes. Make sure all is evenly coated.

Serve on your favorite crackers, pita or bread, adding lettuce if desired. Garnish lavishly with grated carrot and cilantro.

Viola!

This is a simple, delicious meal that is perfect for lunches. This meal fights inflammation because of the high turmeric amount.

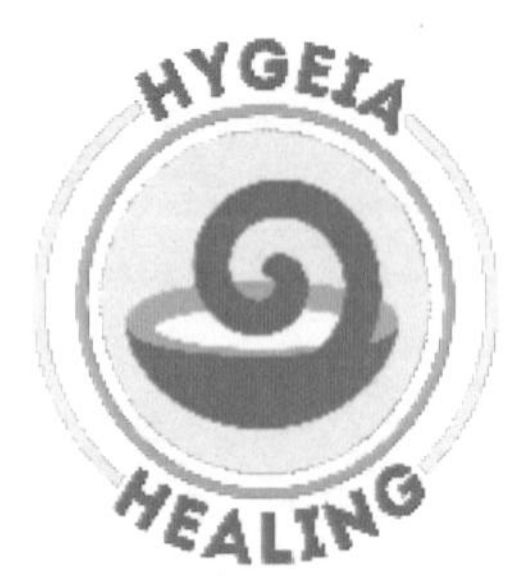

V	E	GG	I	E
Zucchini	Orange	Golden Beets	Grapes	Strawberries
Yellow Squash	Jicama	Purple asparagus	Blackberries	Broccoli
Potato	Cilantro	You Choose ________	Green pepper	Butter Lettuce
Banana	blueberries	Celery	Snap Peas	Apple
Avocado	Carrots	Pineapple	Apricot	Tomatoes

Do not eat items you have an allergy to. Substitute with a different healthy whole fruit or vegetable of your choice.

** Fresh Cilantro may not technically be considered a veggie However it is a green leafy item packed full of vitamins and great for detoxing!*

Spring Week 6

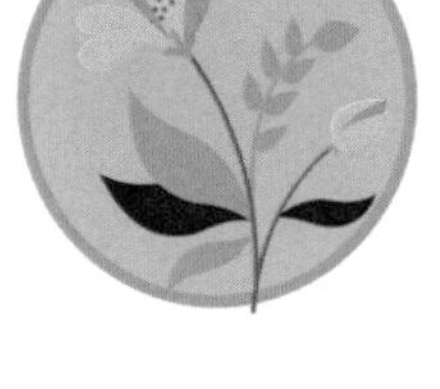

V	E	GG	I	E
Cherries	Broccoli	Green Pepper	Cilantro or Parsley *	Jalapeño
Red Swiss chard	Banana	Nectarine	Carrots	Celery
Green Swiss Chard	Zucchini	You Choose ________	Mushroom	Avocado
Tat soi	Yellow Pepper	Kalamata olives	Apple	Strawberry
Orange	Arugula	Blueberries	Cucumber	Spinach

Do not eat items you have an allergy to. Substitute with a different healthy whole fruit or vegetable of your choice.

** Fresh cilantro or parsley may not technically be considered a veggie However they are green leafy items that are great for cleaning out The GI tract and the liver.*

Spring Week 7

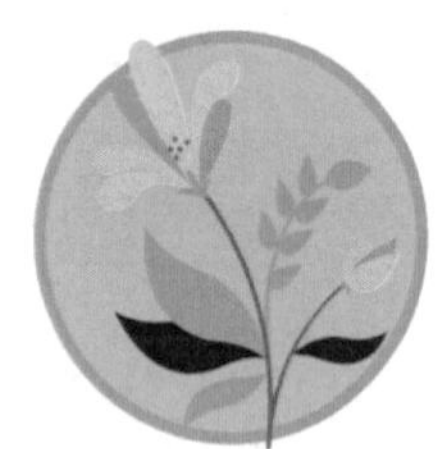

V	E	GG	I	E
Cherries	Broccoli	Green Pepper	Cilantro or Parsley *	Jalapeño
Cauliflower	Banana	Nectarine	Onion	Tomato
Green beans	Zucchini	You Choose ________	Mushroom	Avocado
Rainbow Carrots	Yellow Pepper	Watermelon	Apple	Strawberries
Orange	Purple Cabbage	Blueberries	Edamame	Spinach

Do not eat items you have an allergy to. Substitute with a different healthy whole fruit or vegetable of your choice.
** Fresh cilantro or parsley may not technically be considered a veggie*
However they are green leafy items that are great for cleaning out
The GI tract and the liver.

Spring Week 8

What vegetables do sailors hate?

Leeks!

V	E	GG	I	E
Blackberries	Peaches	Romaine Lettuce	Kiwi	Spinach
Green Onions	Cherry Tomato	Zucchini	Mushrooms	Summer Squash
Green Bell Pepper	Orange Bell Pepper	You Choose ________	Kalamata Olives	Carrots
Artichokes	Green beans	Fresh Basil*	Corn	Broccoli
Cauliflower	Cucumber	Grapefruit	Apple	Banana

Do not eat items you have an allergy to. Substitute with a different healthy whole fruit or vegetable of your choice.
** Fresh Basil may not technically be considered a veggie*
However it is a green leafy item packed full of vitamins and great for detoxing!

Spring Week 9

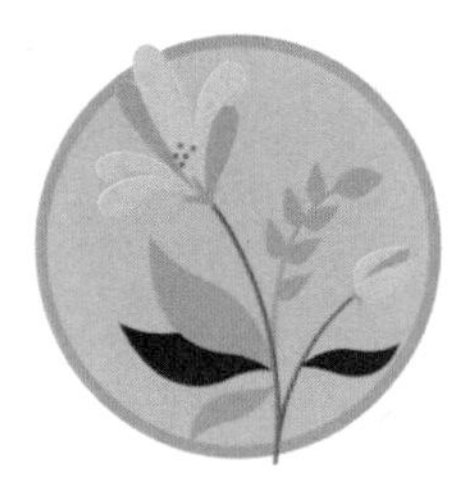

V	E	GG	I	E
Raspberries	Nectarine	Arugula	Avocado	Blueberries
Cucumber	Heirloom Tomatoes	Eggplant	Kohlrabi	Mushrooms
Red Pepper	Shallots	You Choose ________	Jalapeño	Zucchini
Artichokes	Asparagus	Spinach	Bok Choy	Fennel
Radish	Walla Walla onion	Watercress	Orange	Banana

Do not eat items you have an allergy to. Substitute with a different healthy whole fruit or vegetable of your choice.

Spring Week 10

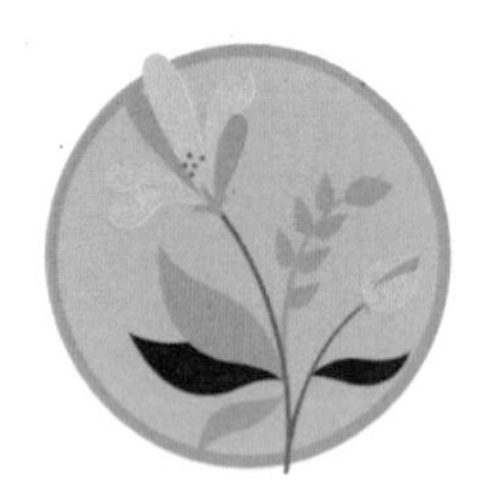

Why don't oysters share their pearls?

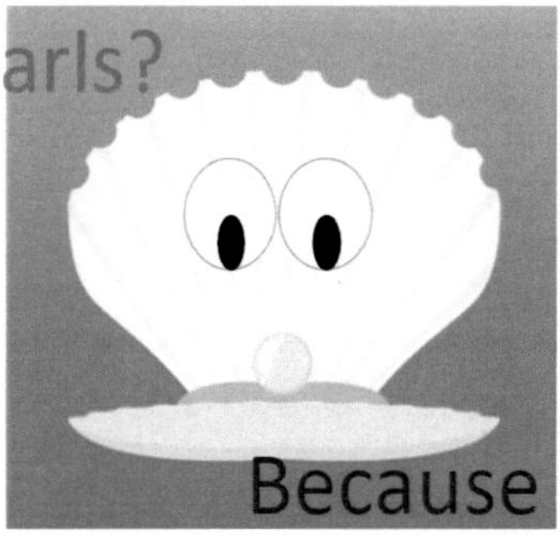

Because they are shellfish!

V	E	GG	I	E
Heirloom Tomatoes	Basil*	Corn	Zucchini	Onion
Eggplant	Jalapeños	Apricot	Cherries	Beets
Blackberries	Blueberries	You Choose ________	Spinach	Kale
Cucumber	Olives	Spaghetti Squash	Limes	Honeydew Melon
Peaches	Strawberries	Watermelon	Butter Lettuce	Green Beans

Do not eat items you have an allergy to. Substitute with a different healthy whole fruit or vegetable of your choice.
** Fresh Basil may not technically be considered a veggie*
However it is a green leafy item packed full of vitamins and great for detoxing!

Spring Week 11

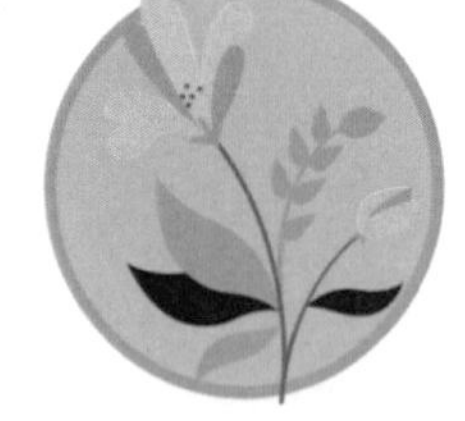

Favorite Morning Shake

Makes 2 servings

Ingredients:

1 cup frozen blueberries

2 cup almond milk

2 cup plain fat-free Greek yogurt

2 handfuls (1/2 cup) walnuts

1 banana

1 large handful spinach

1 tablespoon of ground flax seeds

SHAKE PREPARATION

Put all ingredients in your blender and blend away until completely smooth! If the shake is too thick for your liking, add a little more almond milk. If not thick enough, add a little more yogurt.

This is a great way to get in veggies and a balanced breakfast in the morning.

If you want to really round out this shake and make it follow the Mediterranean Lifestyle, add ½ cup of uncooked rolled oats, blend and enjoy!

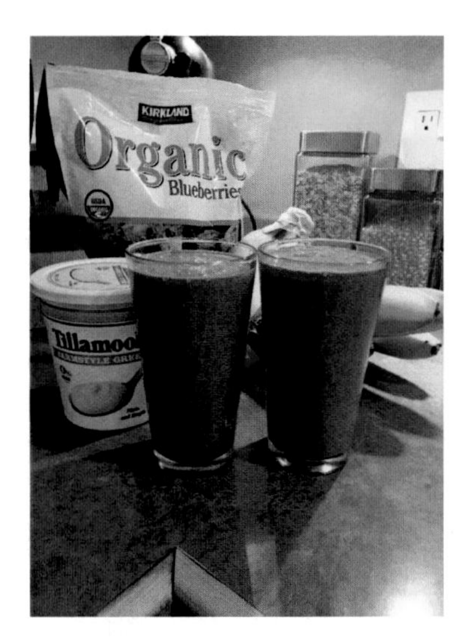

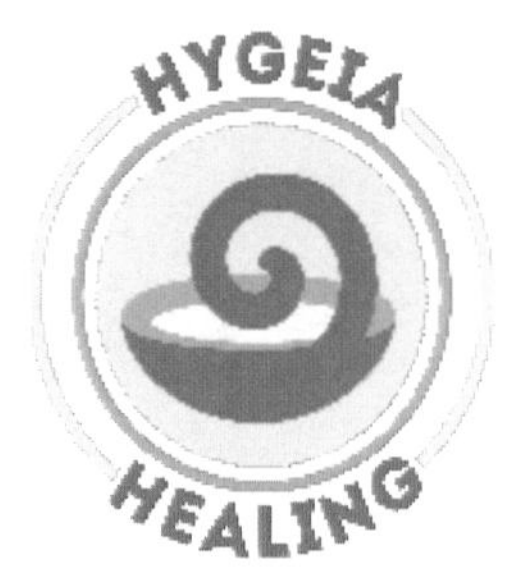

V	E	GG	I	E
Honeydew Melon	Banana	Snow Peas	Broccoli	Green beans
Spaghetti Squash	Romaine	Spinach	Chard	Purple Cabbage
Nectarine	Raspberries	You Choose ________	Beets	Yellow Onion
Zucchini	Cucumber	Tomatoes	Carrots	Strawberries
Basil*	Blackberries	Grapefruit	Apple	Blueberries

Do not eat items you have an allergy to. Substitute with a different healthy whole fruit or vegetable of your choice.

** Fresh Basil may not technically be considered a veggie*
However it is a green leafy item packed full of vitamins and great for detoxing!

Spring Week 12

V	E	GG	I	E
Kalamata Olives	Purple Onions	Asparagus	Peas	Celery
Spaghetti Squash	Artichoke hearts	Bok Choy	Carrots	Blueberries
Spinach	Romaine Lettuce	You Choose ________	Parsnip	Mushrooms
Lemon	Zucchini	Red Pepper	Pear	Orange
Cucumber	Red Potato	Apple	Banana	Butternut squash

Do not eat items you have an allergy to. Substitute with a different healthy whole fruit or vegetable of your choice.

Spring Week 13

V	E	GG	I	E
Tomatoes	Olives	Artichokes	Green Pepper	Mushrooms
Onion	Limes	Grapefruit	Orange	Cherries
Mango	Avocado	You Choose ________	Blueberries	Grapes
Strawberries	Spinach	Banana	Pineapple	Zucchini
Jalapeño	Corn	Cilantro*	Red Pepper	Broccoli

Do not eat items you have an allergy to. Substitute with a different healthy whole fruit or vegetable of your choice.
** Fresh cilantro may not technically be considered a veggie However it is a green leafy item that is great for cleaning out The GI tract and the liver.*

Summer Week 1

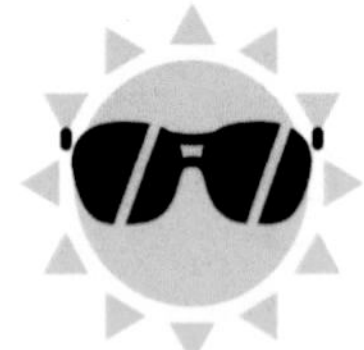

Muff-a-Lotta bowls

Makes 4 Hearty servings

Ingredients:

1 cup Organic Farro

Chicken Stock (3 cups = 1 box) (or Vegetable stock)

Salt & Pepper

2 teaspoonfuls chopped garlic (buy pre-chopped in jar)

2 T olive oil

½ cup chopped flat leaf parsley

1 cup olive tapenade (I love the New Season's prepared olive tapenade, it also has capers! Yum)

2 cup chopped cooked chicken (omit for vegetarian option)

Salt & Pepper

EASY COOKED CHICKEN

In a slow cooker place 3-4 chicken breasts. Add salt & pepper & Italian seasoning herbs to cover. Then add 4 cups chicken stock. Cook on Low for 8 hours or on High for 4 hours. Once cooked, remove from liquid and shred or chop the chicken for use in your favorite dishes.

FARO PREPARATION

To make the faro, in a large pot combine 3 cups of chicken stock and 1 cup farro. Bring to a boil, then cover and simmer for 30 minutes (check with your specific package). Once the liquid is absorbed, sprinkle with ground salt and pepper to taste. (You can also make farro in a rice cooker with water. Use the brown rice setting and it comes out great. Super for time efficiency.)

Set aside to cool.

Once cool, add in the chopped garlic, olive oil, and parsley.

BOWL PREPARATION

I love to make this dish for lunches, so I separate the farro mixture into 4 separate containers.

Then divvy up the chicken and top each bowl with a hearty spoonful of the olive tapenade. Refrigerate your bowls. This dish is best eaten cool.

Makes 4 hearty portions.

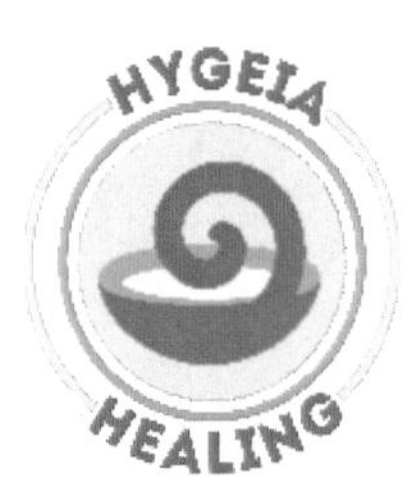

V	E	GG	I	E
Spinach	Blackberries	Avocado	Cilantro or Parsley *	Mango
Pineapple	Banana	Peach	Grapefruit	Zucchini
Nectarine	Cherries	You Choose ________	Green Beans	Bok Choy
Bean Sprouts	Carrots	Snow peas	Cabbage	Lettuce (your choice)
Watercress	Hearts of Palm	Blueberries	Bell pepper	Mushroom

Do not eat items you have an allergy to. Substitute with a different healthy whole fruit or vegetable of your choice.

** Fresh cilantro or parsley may not technically be considered a veggie However they are green leafy items that are great for cleaning out The GI tract and the liver.*

Summer Week 2

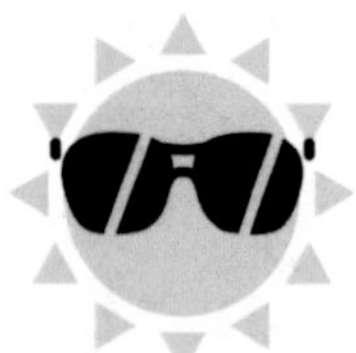

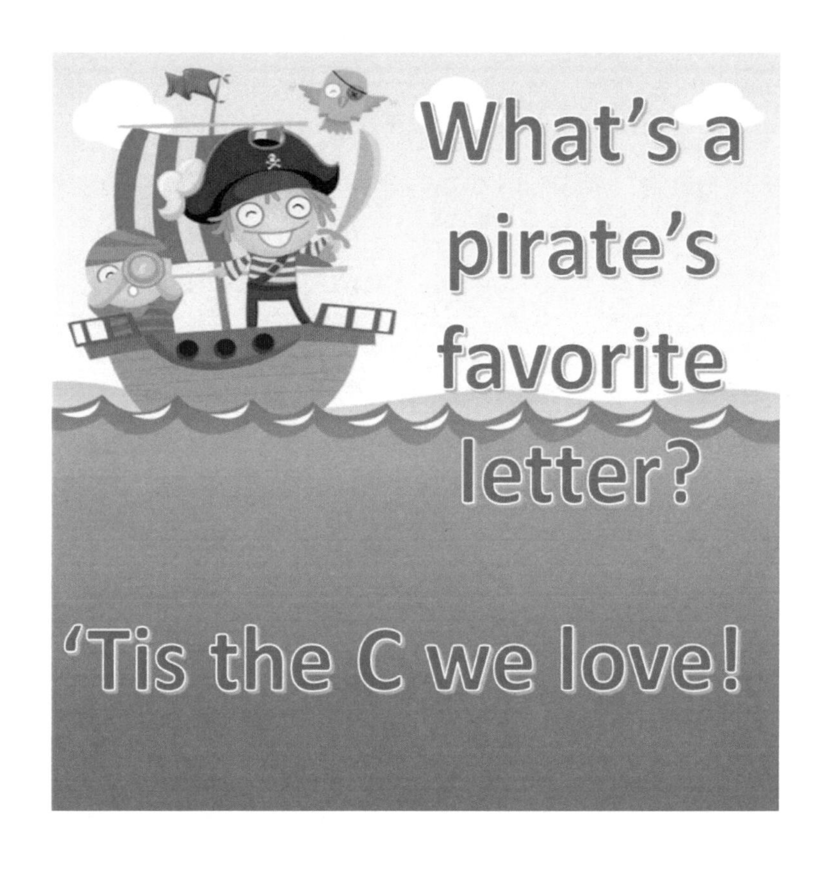
What's a
pirate's
favorite
letter?
'Tis the C we love!

When things are *kinda* rad,
But not totally rad...

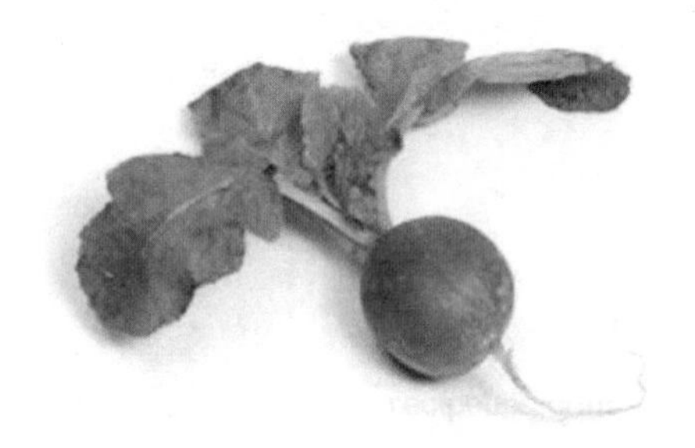

V	E	GG	I	E
Eggplant	Pineapple	Red Pepper	Green Pepper	Mushrooms
Celery	Purple Onion	Green Beans	Snow peas	Edamame
Broccoli	Parsley*	You Choose ________	Yellow Pepper	Carrots
Banana	Blueberries	Kiwi	Zucchini	Bamboo Shoots
Yellow Squash	Cucumber	Orange	Peach	Tomatoes

Do not eat items you have an allergy to. Substitute with a different healthy whole fruit or vegetable of your choice.
** Fresh Parsley may not technically be considered a veggie*
However it is a green leafy item great for cleansing and detoxing!

Summer Week 3

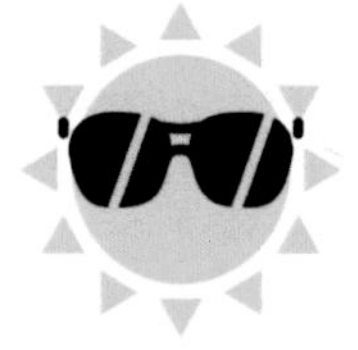

V	E	GG	I	E
Yellow Squash	Peach	Red Pepper	Grapes	Strawberries
Eggplant	Jicama	Asparagus	Blackberries	Peas
Broccoli	Cilantro*	You Choose ________	Green pepper	Celery
Banana	Blueberries	Kiwi	Zucchini	Spinach
Avocado	Carrots	Orange	Peach	Tomatoes

Do not eat items you have an allergy to. Substitute with a different healthy whole fruit or vegetable of your choice.
** Fresh Cilantro may not technically be considered a veggie*
However it is a green leafy item packed full of vitamins and great for detoxing!

Summer Week 4

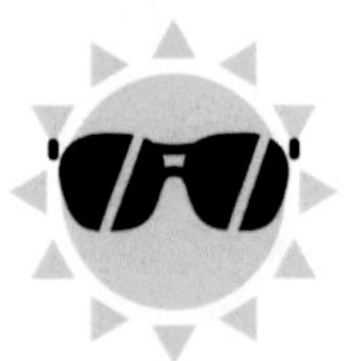

Where does the sun go for a haircut?

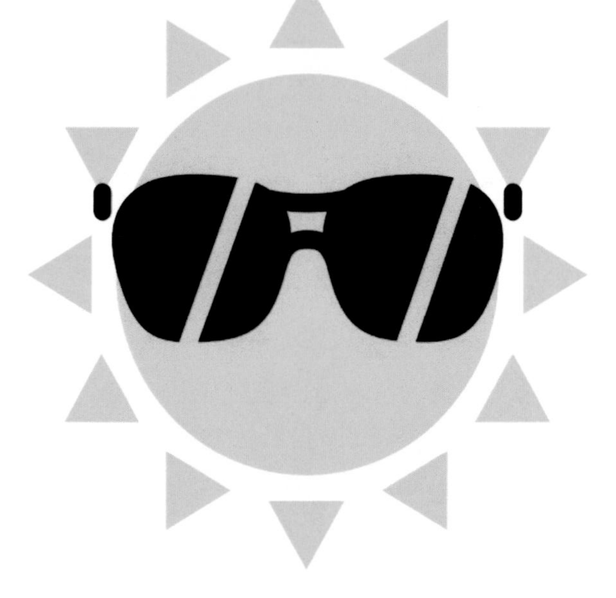

E-Clips!

V	E	GG	I	E
White Onion	Olives	Peach	Peppadew Peppers	Orange
Grapes	Mache Rosettes	Tomatoes	Zucchini	Broccoli
Bok Choy	Raspberries	You Choose ________	Spinach	Kale
Eggplant	Avocado	Carrots	Green beans	Grapefruit
Sprouts	Cucumber	Mango	Blueberries	Corn

Do not eat items you have an allergy to. Substitute with a different healthy whole fruit or vegetable of your choice.

Summer Week 5

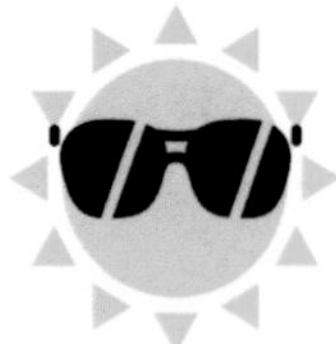

Fruit Salad Shake

Makes 2 servings

Ingredients:

1 cup fruit salad

1 cup almond milk

1 cup plain fat-free Greek yogurt

1 handful (1/4 cup) walnuts

1 Tablespoon Super seeds (or chia)

1 banana

1 large handful spinach

SHAKE PREPARATION

Put all ingredients in your blender and blend away until completely smooth! If the shake is too thick for your liking, add a little more almond milk. If not thick enough, add a little more yogurt.

This is a great way to get in your fruits, veggies and a balanced breakfast in the morning.

Use the Veggie Bingo card for this week to help inspire you in your fruit salad! Make it the night before for a great dessert, then add it for the shake in the morning for breakfast!

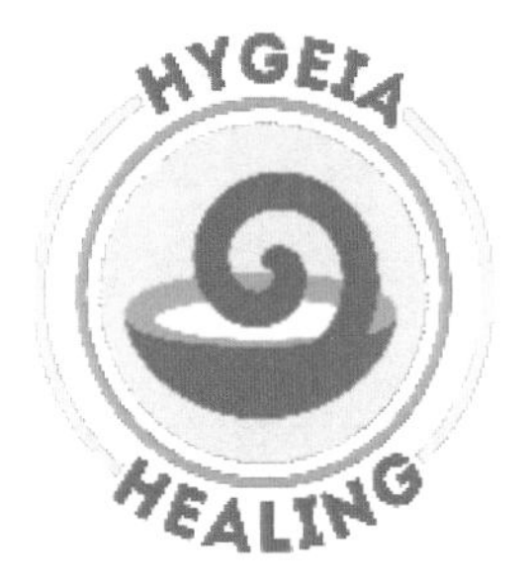

V	E	GG	I	E
Zucchini	Grapefruit	Radicchio	Banana	Raspberries
Yellow Squash	Snow Peas	Watermelon	Cantaloupe	Broccoli
Lemons	Romaine	You Choose ________	Green Pepper	Radish
Red Grapes	Blueberries	Cabbage	Bamboo Shoots	Apple
Avocado	Carrots	Nectarine	Peach	Tomatoes

Do not eat items you have an allergy to. Substitute with a different healthy whole fruit or vegetable of your choice.

Summer Week 6

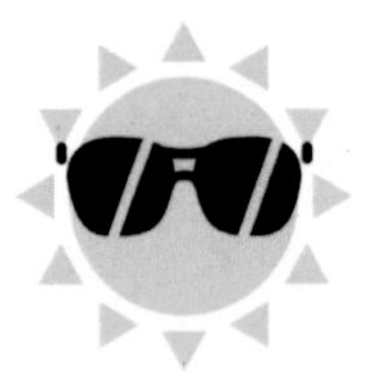

You can't run in
a campground...

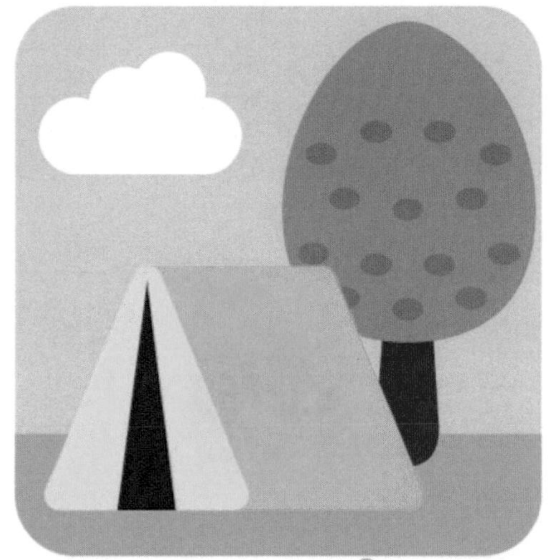

You can only ran,
because it's past tents.

V	E	GG	I	E
Sweet potato	Avocado	Green beans	Broccoli	Green pepper
Yellow Squash	Kale	Spinach	Bok choy	Cabbage
Jalapeño	Mushrooms	You Choose ________	Red pepper	Purple onion
Zucchini	Cucumber	Tomatoes	Carrots	Celery
Cilantro*	Grapes	Orange	Dates	Cherries

Do not eat items you have an allergy to. Substitute with a different healthy whole fruit or vegetable of your choice.

** Fresh Cilantro may not technically be considered a veggie*
However it is a green leafy item packed full of vitamins and great for detoxing!

Summer Week 7

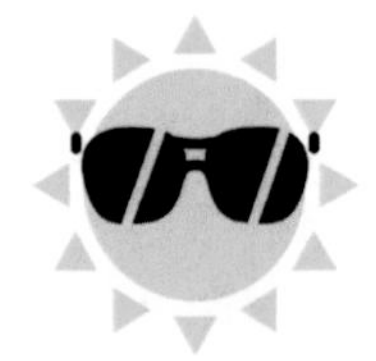

V	E	GG	I	E
Papaya	Banana	Apples	Kiwi	Avocado
Nectarine	Blackberries	Honeydew	Spinach	Portabella Mushrooms
Carrots	Cucumber	You Choose ________	Broccolini	Asparagus
Tomatoes	Onion	Cauliflower	Lemon	Anaheim Pepper
Corn	Zucchini	Romaine Lettuce	Snap Peas	Edamame

Do not eat items you have an allergy to. Substitute with a different healthy whole fruit or vegetable of your choice.

Summer Week 8

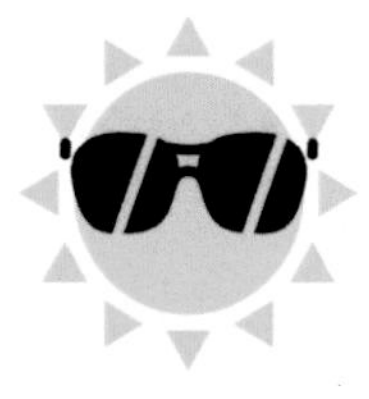

Drunken veggies

Makes 4 big servings

Ingredients:

1 T olive oil

1 T minced garlic

Chopped Veggies I recommend:

Purple onion, mushrooms, red bell pepper, green bell pepper, zucchini, yellow squash, celery, carrots

1 jar organic Vodka Sauce (find it by spaghetti sauces)

Salt & Pepper

Al dente noodles or tortellini of your choice or spaghetti squash

SAUCE PREPARATION

In a large skillet, heat the oil, then add the garlic and chopped veggies. Cook for ~ 5 minutes with the lid on stirring occasionally, until at the level of doneness you prefer. Add in the entire jar of vodka sauce and heat until bublling.

PUTTING IT TOGETHER

If you are using pasta, cook via directions on the package. If using spaghetti squash, split the squash into halves, lengthwise, remove seeds. Microwave each half for ~10 minutes until hot and tender. Use a fork to scrape the flesh out of the rind, it will come out like spaghetti.

Serve in bowls, with veggie sauce on top of your pasta or squash.

Enjoy!

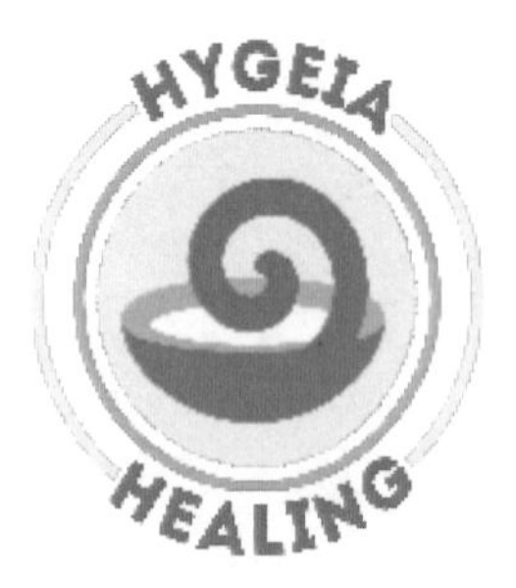

V	E	GG	I	E
Kiwi	Avocado	Jalapeño	Green Beans	Cauliflower
Spinach	Arugula	Green Onion	Purple Onion	Tomato
Yellow Pepper	Zucchini	You Choose ________	Lemons	Broccolini
Carrots	Strawberry	Asparagus	Bananas	Watermelon
Kale	Bok Choy	Blueberries	Pineapple	Corn

Do not eat items you have an allergy to. Substitute with a different healthy whole fruit or vegetable of your choice.

Summer Week 9

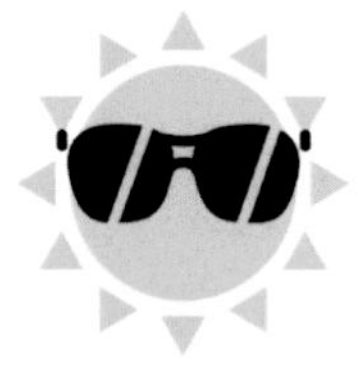

V	E	GG	I	E
Peach	Cherries	Green Chilies	Jicama	Brussel Sprouts
Spinach	Arugula	Green Onion	Yellow Onion	Banana
Red Pepper	Apple	You Choose ________	Limes	Kale
Green beans	Cucumber	Broccoli	Tomatoes	Watermelon
Chard	Avocado	Radish	Romaine	Corn

Do not eat items you have an allergy to. Substitute with a different healthy whole fruit or vegetable of your choice.

Summer Week 10

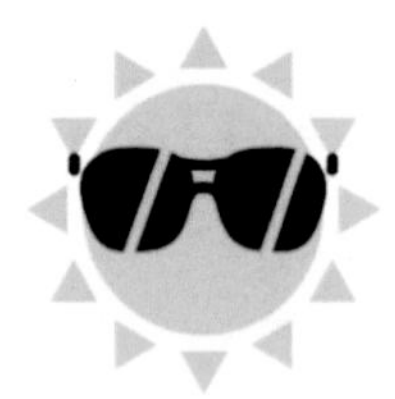

Greek Salad

Makes 4-6 servings

Ingredients:

1 cup Orzo

½ cup chopped walnuts or toasted pine nuts

The juice of 2 fresh lemons

3 T olive oil

1 cup Kalamata olives (drained)

1 chopped red pepper

1 chopped cucumber

1 cup chopped purple onion

½ cup chopped fresh flat leaf parsley

1 cup sliced cherry tomatoes

1 cup crumbled feta cheese

Pepper to taste

ORZO PREPARATION

Boil salted water and cook the orzo for 9 minutes (or per package directions). Drain and rinse with cold water.

Set aside.

BOWL PREPARATION

Put all ingredients in large bowl, including cooled orzo. Mix well to combine.

Makes 4-6 servings.

This is a refreshing salad that can be a side dish or a main dish. The olives and feta have a great salty taste so additional salt is not needed. Great for a hot day!

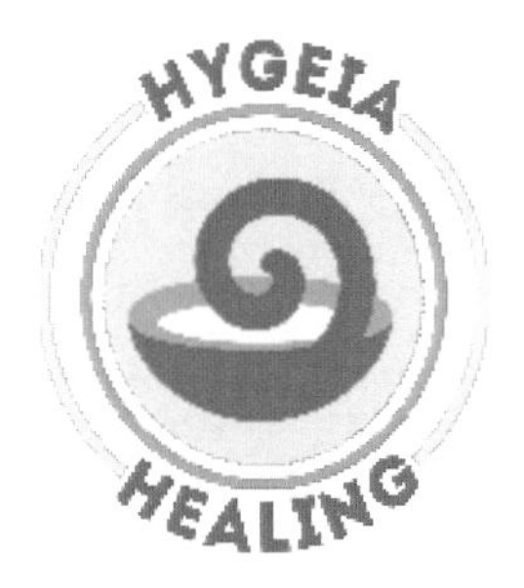

V	E	GG	I	E
Strawberry	Kiwi	Cantaloupe	Fresh mint and/or cilantro*	Nectarine
Apple	Banana	Pluot	Grapes	Orange
Black olives	Green onion	You Choose ________	Purple onion	Avocado
Celery	Jalapeno	Corn	Green pepper	Yellow pepper
Spinach	Carrots	Blueberries	Cucumber	Summer squash

Do not eat items you have an allergy to. Substitute with a different healthy whole fruit or vegetable of your choice.
** Fresh mint & cilantro may not technically be considered a veggie However they are green leafy items that are great for cleaning out The GI tract and the liver.*

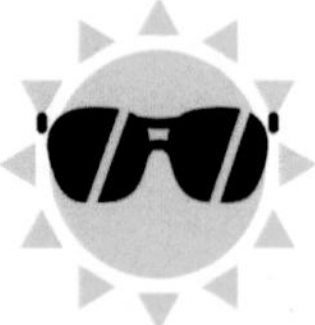

Summer Week 11

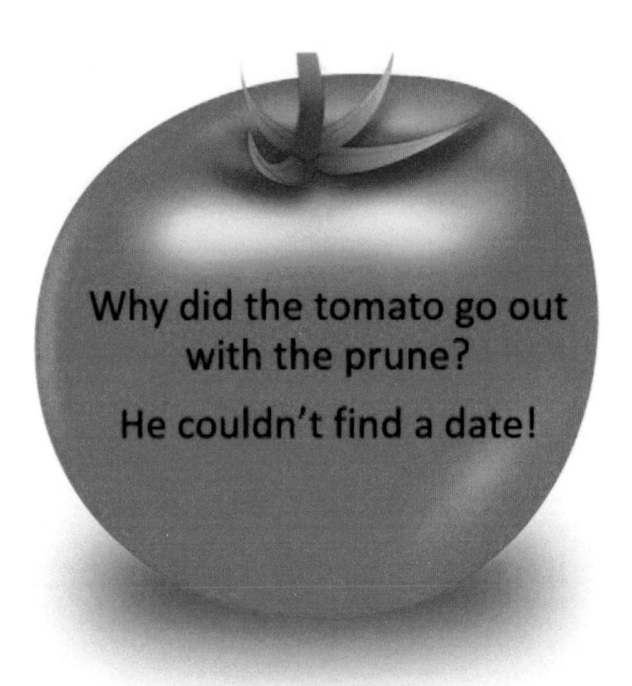
Why did the tomato go out with the prune?
He couldn't find a date!

V	E	GG	I	E
Tomatoes	Avocado	Jalapeño	Green Beans	Cauliflower
Spinach	Red Leaf Lettuce	Green Onion	Purple Onion	Asparagus
Yellow Pepper	Zucchini	You Choose ________	Lemons	Broccoli
Carrots	Sweet Potato	Celery	Bananas	Olives
Kale	Bok Choy	Blueberries	Raspberries	Apples

Do not eat items you have an allergy to. Substitute with a different healthy whole fruit or vegetable of your choice.

Summer Week 12

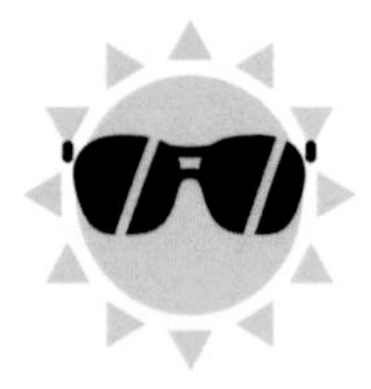

Carrot Delight shake

Makes 2 servings

Ingredients:

1 cup carrot juice

1 cup almond milk

1 cup plain fat-free Greek yogurt

1 handful (1/4 cup) walnuts

1 Tablespoon Super seeds (or ground flax seeds)

1 banana

1 large handful spinach

SHAKE PREPARATION

Put all ingredients in your blender and blend away until completely smooth! If the shake is too thick for your liking, add a little more almond milk. If not thick enough, add a little more yogurt.

This is a great way to get in veggies and a balanced breakfast in the morning.

Total calories if using the ingredients pictured is ~330, protein 15 grams, sugars 15 grams in each serving.

In this particular version I used a carrot + orange + ginger juice so the shake has a bit of spice and more sugar than just plain carrot juice.

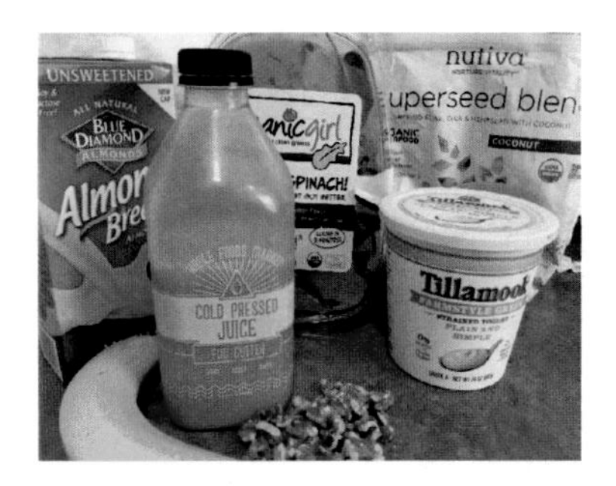

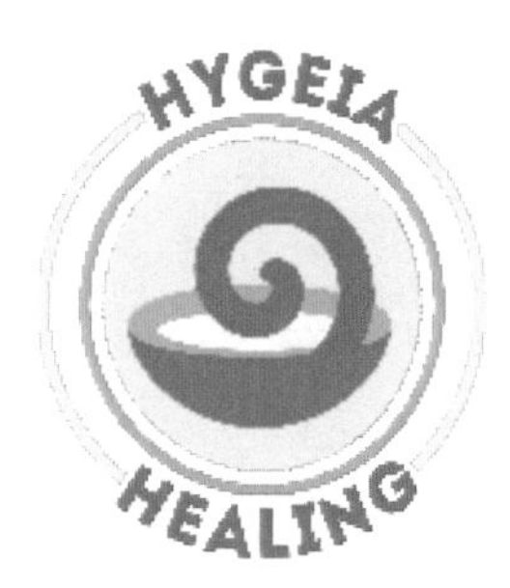

V	E	GG	I	E
Asparagus	Yellow Onions	Parsley*	Peas	Celery
Pineapple	Artichoke hearts	Kale	Carrots	Blueberries
Spinach	Romaine Lettuce	You Choose ________	Cabbage	Mushrooms
Lemon	Zucchini	Brussel Sprouts	Apple	Kiwi
Green Beans	Banana Peppers	Grapes	Banana	Butternut squash

Do not eat items you have an allergy to. Substitute with a different healthy whole fruit or vegetable of your choice.
** Fresh parsley may not technically be considered a veggie However it is a green leafy item that is great for cleaning out the GI tract and the liver.*

Summer Week 13

V	E	GG	I	E
Mango	Avocado	Jalapeño	Green Beans	Cauliflower
Spinach	Red Leaf Lettuce	Green Onion	Purple Onion	Tomato
Yellow Pepper	Zucchini	You Choose ________	Lemons	Broccolini
Carrots	Parsnip	Asparagus	Banana	Orange (or cutie)
Kale	Bok Choy	Blueberries	Pumpkin	Corn

Do not eat items you have an allergy to. Substitute with a different healthy whole fruit or vegetable of your choice.

Autumn Week 1

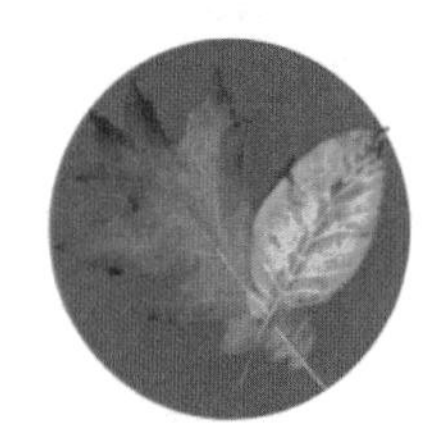

Butternut Squash Pasta

MAKES 4 SERVINGS

Ingredients

2 T olive oil

1 T chopped garlic

1 peeled, seeded and chopped butternut squash

½ cup water

1/3 cup chopped white onion

Salt & Pepper to taste

2-3T more olive oil

2 T fresh sage, chopped

Fresh fettuccini pasta

Fresh grated parmesan cheese (optional)

In large skillet sauté the olive oil, garlic and butternut squash for 5 minutes. Add ½ cup water to pan, cover and simmer until the squash is tender (~10-15 minutes).

Add the chopped white onion, salt and pepper, extra olive oil and fresh sage. Sauté another 5 minutes or so until the onion is tender.

Serve over your fresh cooked pasta and garnish with a little parmesan cheese. Delish!

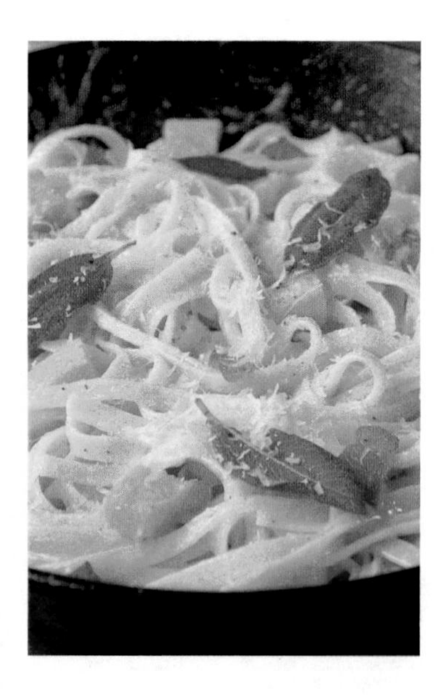

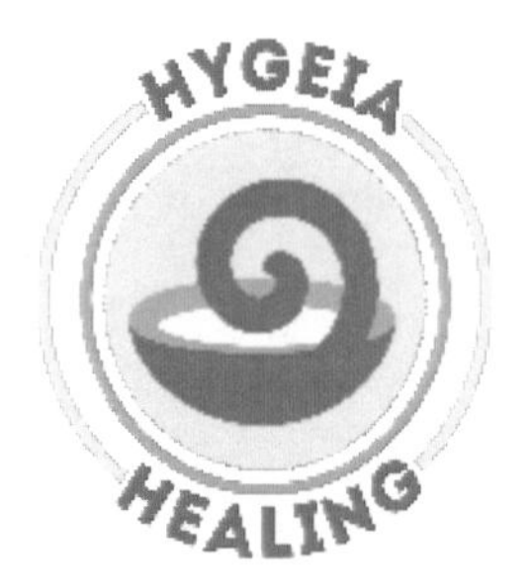

V	E	GG	I	E
Mango	Avocado	Jalapeño	Green Beans	Cauliflower
Spinach	Red Leaf Lettuce	Green Onion	Purple Onion	Tomato
Yellow Pepper	Zucchini	You Choose ________	Lemons	Broccolini
Carrots	Parsnip	Asparagus	Bananas	Orange (or cutie)
Kale	Bok Choy	Blueberries	Pumpkin	Corn

Do not eat items you have an allergy to. Substitute with a different healthy whole fruit or vegetable of your choice.

Autumn Week 2

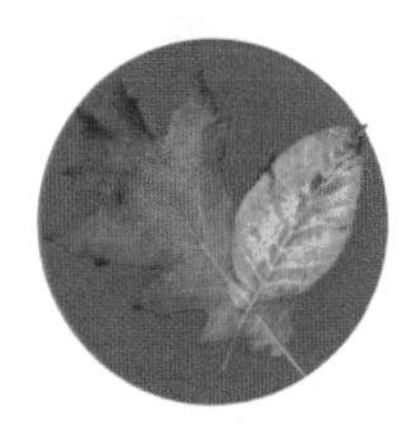

V	E	GG	I	E
Grapes	Broccoli	Green Pepper	Cilantro or Parsley *	Peppadew Pepper
Cauliflower	Banana	Apple	Onion	Tomato
Green beans	Zucchini	You Choose ________	Mushroom	Avocado
Rainbow Carrots	Yellow Pepper	Cucumber	Cucumber	Celery
Orange or cutie	Peas	Blueberries	Sweet Potato	Spinach

Do not eat items you have an allergy to. Substitute with a different healthy whole fruit or vegetable of your choice.
** Fresh cilantro or parsley may not technically be considered a veggie However they are green leafy items that are great for cleaning out The GI tract and the liver.*

Autumn Week 3

Why do fungi have
to pay double bus fares?

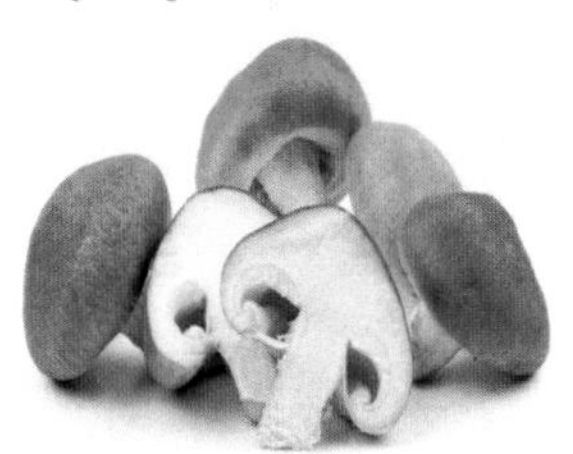

Because they take up too mushroom!

V	E	GG	I	E
Tomatoes	Olives	Potato	Green Pepper	Mushrooms
Onion	Carrots	Parsnip	Orange	Apple
Kale	Avocado	You Choose ________	Blueberries	Grapes
Celery	Spinach	Banana	Beets	Zucchini
Delicata Squash	Corn	Cilantro*	Red Pepper	Broccoli

Do not eat items you have an allergy to. Substitute with a different healthy whole fruit or vegetable of your choice.
** Fresh cilantro may not technically be considered a veggie However it is a green leafy item that is great for cleaning out The GI tract and the liver.*

Autumn Week 4

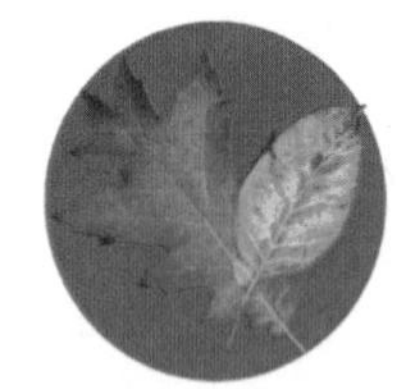

What does a vegan zombie eat?

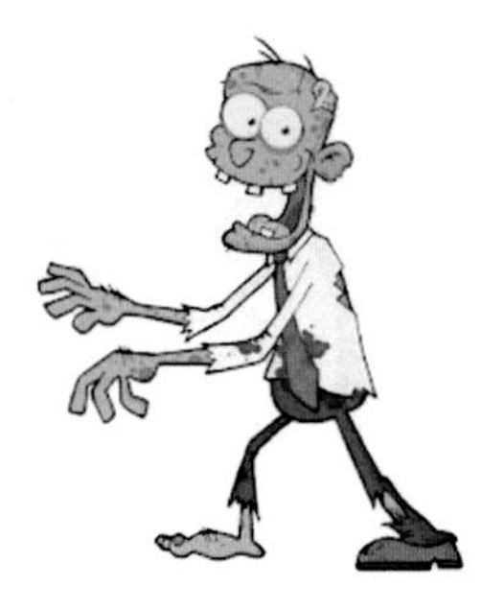

Graaaaaaaaaaains!

V	E	GG	I	E
Arugula	Artichoke Hearts	Asparagus	Bok Choy	Banana
Beets	Cabbage	Carrots	Chard	Spinach
Mushrooms	Apples	You Choose ________	Blueberries	Pumpkin
Purple Onion	Celery	Jalapeño	Green beans	Peas
Zucchini	Yellow Squash	Spaghetti Squash	Pear	Red Potato

Do not eat items you have an allergy to. Substitute with a different healthy whole fruit or vegetable of your choice.

Autumn Week 5

V	E	GG	I	E
Kalamata Olives	Artichoke Hearts	Green Beans	Parsley*	Blackberries
Zucchini	Broccoli	Carrots	Tomato	Spinach
Banana	Apples	You Choose ________	Blueberries	Pumpkin or Delicata Squash
Purple Onion	Celery	Jalapeño	Cabbage	Peas
Kale	Orange	Mushrooms	Pear	Red Potato

Do not eat items you have an allergy to. Substitute with a different healthy whole fruit or vegetable of your choice.

** Fresh parsley may not technically be considered a veggie However it is a green leafy item that is great for cleaning out The GI tract and the liver.*

Autumn Week 6

V	E	GG	I	E
Apple	Avocado	Green Pepper	Squash of your choosing!	Leeks
Corn	Banana	Cabbage	Purple Onion	Tomato
Kale	Zucchini	You Choose ________	Mushroom	Broccoli
Carrots	Red Pepper	Cucumber	Radish	Grapefruit
Celery	Asparagus	Blueberries	Romaine lettuce	Spinach

Do not eat items you have an allergy to. Substitute with a different healthy whole fruit or vegetable of your choice.

Autumn Week 7

Tex Mex Chowder

Ingredients

3 Tablespoons olive oil

3 stalks celery - chopped

1 medium white onion - chopped

1 small purple onion - chopped

1 medium can diced green chilies

1 Tablespoon chili powder

Salt & Pepper to taste

1 teaspoonful Italian herb seasoning

2 carrots - chopped

1 red bell pepper - chopped

1 green bell pepper - chopped

1 medium zucchini - chopped

handful of cilantro - chopped

1 can diced tomatoes in juice

2 cans rinsed black beans

1 can rinsed corn

1 cup quinoa

1-2 cups shredded roasted turkey (omit for vegetarian option)

2 boxes (8 cups) chicken or vegetable stock

1 cup shredded cheddar or jalapeño jack cheese (omit for vegan option)

1 avocado - sliced

Tortilla chips

MAKES 10 SERVINGS

In large stock pot, sauté the olive oil, onions, and green chilies. Add in the seasonings and sauté for about 5-6 minutes until onions just start getting tender. Add in carrots, celery and bell peppers, sauté another 3-4 minutes. Add in the zucchini, cilantro, tomatoes, black beans, corn, turkey, quinoa and chicken stock. Bring to a boil, then cover and simmer for 15 minutes. Taste the soup and add more seasonings to your liking. Simmer another 15 minutes, until the quinoa is cooked (it opens into a circle). Ladle into soup bowls and stir in a small handful of cheese, this makes it creamy and delicious. Serve with tortilla chips and avocado as a garnish.

Enjoy!

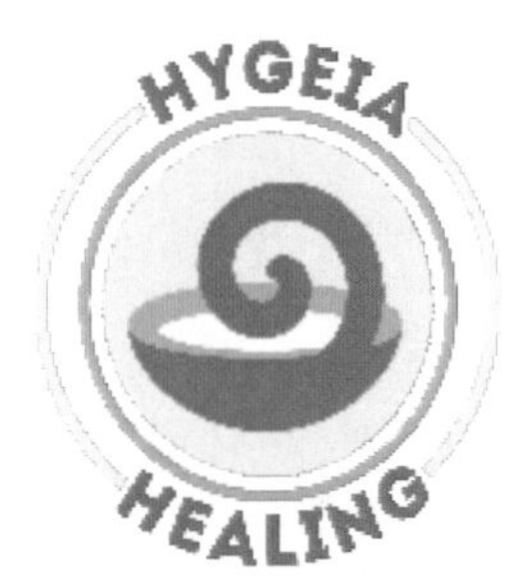

V	E	GG	I	E
Orange or cutie	Apple	Banana	Blueberries	Mango
Strawberry	Blackberry	Avocado	Cabbage	Cherry tomatoes
Green Onions	Green Bell Pepper	You Choose ________	Zucchini	Olives
Broccoli	Corn	Jalapeño	Corn	Cilantro*
Grapefruit	Fennel	Arugula	Romaine Lettuce	Red Potato

Do not eat items you have an allergy to. Substitute with a different healthy whole fruit or vegetable of your choice.
** Fresh cilantro may not technically be considered a veggie However it is a green leafy item that is great for cleaning out The GI tract and the liver.*

Autumn Week 8

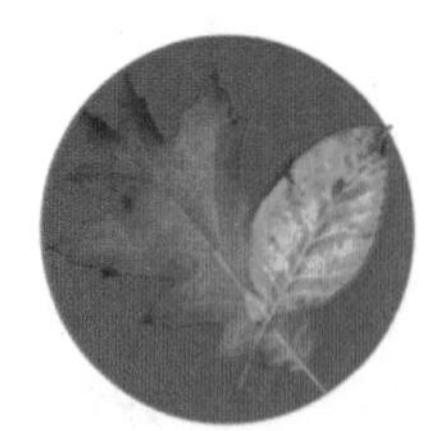

V	E	GG	I	E
Peas	Apple	Banana	Blueberries	Strawberry
Grapefruit	Mango	Avocado	Kale	Green beans
Purple Onion	Red Bell Pepper	You Choose ________	Zucchini	Olives
Broccoli	Corn	Green chilies	Mushrooms	Parsley*
Potato	Cauliflower	Spinach	Olives	Butternut squash

Do not eat items you have an allergy to. Substitute with a different healthy whole fruit or vegetable of your choice.

** Fresh parsley may not technically be considered a veggie*
However it is a green leafy item that is great for cleaning out
The GI tract and the liver.

Autumn Week 9

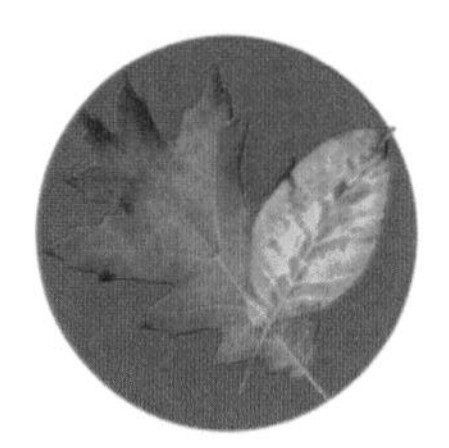

How do you make a skeleton laugh?

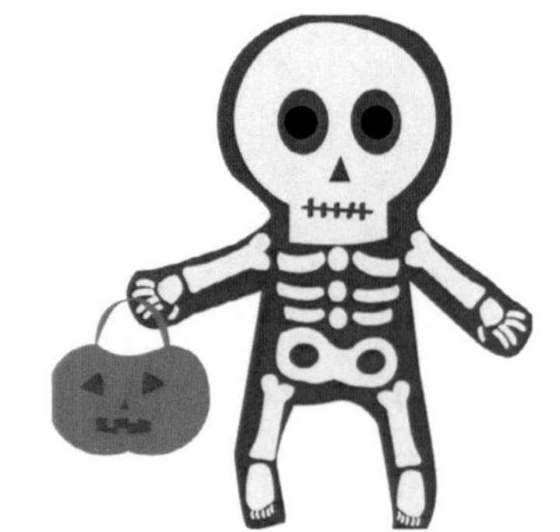

Tickle his funny bone!

V	E	GG	I	E
Lemon	Red Pepper	Red onion	Cilantro*	Tomato
Yellow squash	Zucchini	Butternut squash	Potato	Peas
Mache Rosettes	Tomatillos	You Choose ________	Lime	Parsley*
Corn	Avocado	Butter Lettuce	Broccoli	Kale
Edamame	Carrots	Spinach	Artichoke	Green Onion

Do not eat items you have an allergy to. Substitute with a different healthy whole fruit or vegetable of your choice.

** Fresh basil, cilantro and parsley may not technically be considered veggies, However they are green leafy items that are great for cleaning out The GI tract and the liver.*

Autumn Week 10

V	E	GG	I	E
Mache Rosettes	Broccoli	Green Pepper	Cilantro or Parsley *	Jalapeño
Red Swiss chard	Banana	Nectarine	Carrots	Celery
Green Swiss chard	Zucchini	You Choose ________	Mushroom	Avocado
Tat soi	Yellow Pepper	Kalamata olives	Apple	Artichoke Hearts
Orange	Arugula	Blueberries	Cucumber	Spinach

Do not eat items you have an allergy to. Substitute with a different healthy whole fruit or vegetable of your choice.

** Fresh cilantro or parsley may not technically be considered a veggie However they are green leafy items that are great for cleaning out The GI tract and the liver.*

Autumn Week 11

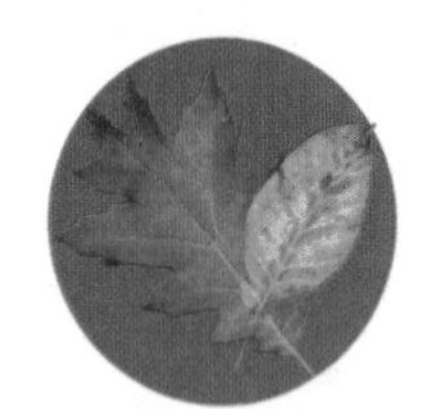

What did the turkey say on Thanksgiving?

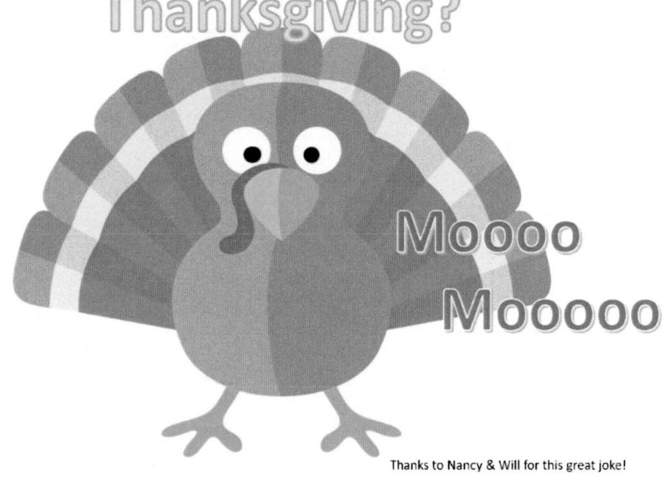

Thanks to Nancy & Will for this great joke!

V	E	GG	I	E
Peach	Broccoli	Green Pepper	Cilantro or Parsley *	Arugula
Mango	Banana	Apple	Onion	Tomato
Green Onions	Zucchini	You Choose ________	Butternut Squash	Celery
Rainbow Carrots	Yellow Pepper	Cucumber	Mache Rosettes	Bok Choy
Orange or cutie	Olives	Blueberries	Sweet potato	Spinach

Do not eat items you have an allergy to. Substitute with a different healthy whole fruit or vegetable of your choice.
*** Fresh cilantro or parsley may not technically be considered a veggie However they are green leafy items that are great for cleaning out The GI tract and the liver.*

Autumn Week 12

V	E	GG	I	E
Radish	Red Leaf Lettuce	Grapefruit	Parsley*	Artichoke
Kumquats	Pineapple	Carrot	Celery	Orange
Spinach	Bok Choy	You Choose ________	Spinach	Pear
Asparagus	Scallions	Leek	Banana	Mushrooms
Butternut Squash	Kalamata Olives	Purple Onion	Jalapeño	Grapes

Do not eat items you have an allergy to. Substitute with a different healthy whole fruit or vegetable of your choice.

** Fresh parsley may not technically be considered a veggie However it is a green leafy item that is great for cleaning out The GI tract and the liver.*

Autumn Week 13

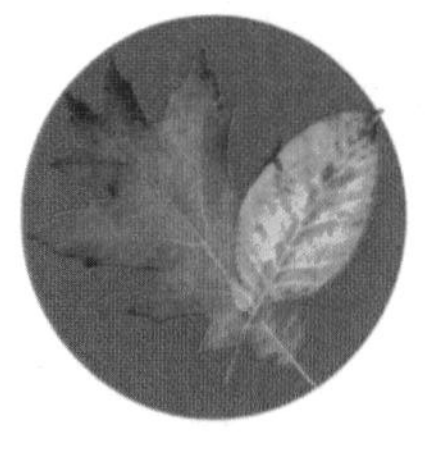

References:

All Jokes have been told to me by clients or come from the website Top 100 Veggie Jokes which can be accessed at: http://secretseedsociety.com/2011/04/27/top-100-veggie-jokes-of-all-time/

All recipes are original Christine Mayo Powers creations except Dori's Tortellini Soup which is an original creation of Dori Hamilton.

All graphics created with the help from Canva.com except photos provided by Lisa Talirico ©2018 ifonfolio.com.

Babio N, et al. Mediterranean diets and metabolic syndrome status in the PREDIMED randomized trial. CMAJ. 2014; DOI:10.1503/cmaj.14074

Banal DK, Ju FB. Effects of walnut consumption on blood lipids and other cardiovascular risk factors: a meta-analysis and systematic review. Am J Clin Nutr. 2009;90(1):56-63.

Blackburn H. Overview: The Seven Countries Study in brief. University of Minnesota, School of Public Health. 2013.

Buchner FL, et al. Variety in fruit and vegetable consumption and risk of lung cancer in the European prospective investigation into cancer and nutrition. Cancer Epidemiol Biomarkers Prev. 2010 Sep; 19(9):2278-86.

Cortes B, et al. Acute effects of high-fat meals enriched with walnuts or olive oil on postprandial endothelial function. J Am Coll Cardiol. 2006;48:1666-1671.

Dala-Vita A, Ros E. Mounting evidence that increased consumption of alpha-linolenic acid, the vegetable omega 3 fatty acid may benefit cardiovascular health. Clin Lipidology. 2011;6(4):365-369.

de Lorgeril M, et al. Mediterranean diet, traditional risk factors and the rate of cardiovascular complications after myocardial infarction. Final report of the Lyon Diet Heart Study. Circulation 1999;99:779-785.

de Lorgeril M, et al. Mediterranean dietary pattern in a randomized trial. prolonged survival and possible reduced cancer rate. Arch Intern med. 1998;158:1181-1187.

Esposito K, et al. Mediterranean diet and weight loss; meta-analysis of randomized controlled trials. metab Syndr relat Disord. 2011;9:1-12.

Estruch R, et al. Primary prevention of cardiovascular disease with Mediterranean diet. N Eng J Med. 2013; 368:1279-1290.

Gadgil MD, et al. The effects of carbohydrate, unsaturated fat, and protein intake on measures of insulin sensitivity: results from the OmniHeart Trial. Diabetes Care. 2013 May;36(5):1132-7.

Gardener H, et al. Mediterranean diet and white matter hyperintensity volume in the Northern Manhattan Study. Arch Neuro. 2012;69(2):251-256.

Guigliano D, Esposito K. Mediterraneandiet and meabolic diseases. Curr Opin Lipidol. 2008;19:63-68.

Harlan TS. The Mediterranean Diet. www.drgourmet.commediterraneandiet/research.shtml

Holt EM, et al. Fruit and vegetable consumption and its relation to markers of inflammation and oxidative stress in adolescents. J Am Diet Assoc. 2009Mar;109(3):414-421.

Howard ME. Living to be 100: 16 Common Lifestyle Characteristics of the Oldest and Healthiest People in the World. Concord, CA: Biomed General, 2017

Jiang Y, et al. Cruciferous vegetable intake is inversely correlated with circulating levels of proinflammatory markers in women. J Acad Nut Det. 2014 May;114(5):700-8.

Kastorini CM, et al. Adherence to the Mediterranean diet in relation to an acute coronary syndrome or stroke nonfatal events: a comparative analysis of case/control study. Am Heart J. 2011;162(4):717-724.

Kastorini CM, et al. The effect of Mediterranean diet on metabolic syndrome and its components: a meta-analysis of 50 studies and 534906 individuals. J Am Coll Cardiol. 2011;57:1299-1313.

Keys A. Mediterranean diet and public health: personal reflections. Am J Clin Nutr. 1995;61(6):1321S-1323S.

Keys A, et al. The diet and 15-year death rate in the Seven Countries Study. Am J Epidemiol. 1986;124:903-915.

Klapcinska B, et al. Antioxidant defenses in centenarians (A preliminary study), Acta Biochem Pol. 2000;47(2):281-292.

Olubukola A, et al. Systematic review and meta-analysis of different dietary approaches to the management of type 2 diabetes. Am J Clin Nutr. 2013;97(3):505-516.

Perls TT, Silver MH, Laureman JF. Living to 100: Lessons in Living to your Maximum Potential at Any Age. New York, NY: Basic Books, 1999.

Tourlouki E, et al. The 'secrets' of the long livers in Mediterranean islands: The MEDIS study. Eur Jour Pub Health. 2009; doi:10.1093/eurpub/ckp192.

Rink SM, et al. Self-report of fruit and vegetable intake that meets the 5 a day recommendation is associated with reduced levels of oxidative stress biomarkers and increased levels of antioxidant defense in premenopausal women. J Acad Nutr Diet. 2013 Jun;113(6):776-85.

Schwingshakl L, Hoffman G. Adherence to Mediterranean diet and risk of cancer: a systematic review and meta-analysis of observational studies. Int J Cancer. 2014;135(8):1884-1897.

Schwingshakl L et al. Adherence to a Mediterranean diet and risk of diabetes: a systematic review and meta-analysis. Pub health Nutr. 2015 May;18(7):1292-9.

Sofi F, et al. Accruing evidence on benefits of adherence to the Mediterranean diet on health: an updated systematic review and meta-analysis. Am J Clin Nutr. 2010;92:1189-1196.

St. Charles A, The Mediterranean Diet: an Approach to Better Health. 2015: June 2nd Ed. Institute for Natural Resources.

Trichopoulou A et al. Conformity to traditional Mediterranean diet and breast cancer risk. Am J Clin Nutr. 2010;92(3):620-625.

Watzl B. Anti-inflammatory effects of plant-based foods and of their constituents. Int J Vitam Nutr Res. 2008 Dec;78(6):293-8.

Willett WC. Eat, Drink and Be Healthy. New York, NY: Free Press, 2001.

About the Author

Dr. Christine Mayo Powers is a board-certified pharmacotherapy specialist and clinical pharmacist who is recognized as a teacher of both Western and Eastern philosophies, specializing in Aging at The Ohio State University. She has trained and become certified in Eden Energy Medicine, Fascial Stretch Therapy and is a Clinical Hypnotherapist offering a transpersonal approach to healing and personal development.

During her career, Dr. Mayo Powers has been on the Nutritional Metabolic Support Team and the Intensive Care Team at local acute care hospitals, worked at mental health and addiction hospitals, and opened her own Healing and Wellness clinic providing preventative care in Portland, Oregon. She currently provides workshops and individual care on aging well, physical functionality, prevention and reversal of common chronic illnesses.

Dr. Mayo Powers currently resides in Oregon seeing clients at her clinic, Hygeia Healing, and also at her online clinic seeing clients all over the world at **takechargeofmyhealth.online**.